Better Health Through Natural Supplements

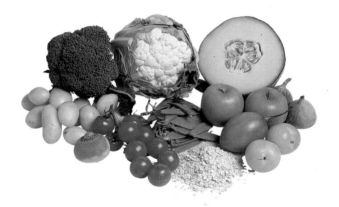

John Briffa, M.D.

B.Sc., M.B., B.S. (London)

TIME
LIFE
BOOKS

Alexandria, Virginia

Time-Life Books is a division of Time Life Inc.

TIME LIFE INC.

PRESIDENT AND CEO: George Artandi

TIME-LIFE CUSTOM PUBLISHING

Vice President and Publisher	Terry Newell
Vice President of Sales and Marketing	Neil Levin
Director of Acquisitions and Editorial Resources	Jennifer Pearce
Director of Creative Services	Laura Ciccone McNeill
Director of Special Markets	Liz Ziehl
Project Manager	Jennie Halfant

Note

Every effort has been taken to ensure that all information in this book is correct and compatible with national standards generally accepted at the time of publication. This book is not intended to replace consultation with your doctor or other healthcare professional. The author and publisher disclaim any liability, loss, injury or damage incurred as a consequence, directly or indirectly, of the use and application of the contents of this book.

First printing. Printed in China

TIME-LIFE is a trademark of Time Warner Inc. U.S.A.
Books produced by Time-Life Custom Publishing are available at a special bulk discount for promotional and premium use. Custom adaptations can also be created to meet your specific marketing goals. Call 1-800-323-5255.

Library of Congress Cataloging-in-Publication Data

Briffa, John.
    Better health through natural supplements / John Briffa.
       p. cm. -- (Time-Life health factfiles)
    ISBN 0-7370-1612-4 (spiral softcover. : alk. paper)
    1. Dietry supplements Popular works. 2. Nutrition Popular works.
3. Orthomolecular therapy Popular works. I. Title. II. Series.
RA784.B6968   1999
613.2'85--dc21   99-27421
                                                          CIP

A Marshall Edition
Conceived, edited and designed by
Marshall Editions
161 New Bond Street
London W1Y 9PA

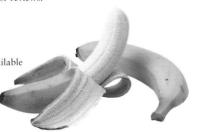

CONTENTS

Everyday Health

Skin and Eyes

Muscles, Bones, and Teeth

The Immune System

Blood, Hormones, and Metabolism

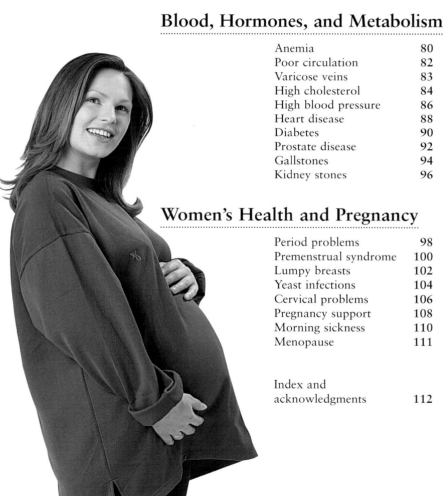

Women's Health and Pregnancy

INTRODUCTION

It is a widely held belief that additional vitamins, minerals, and other nutritional supplements are unnecessary if you eat sensibly. However, while a healthy diet will almost always form the backbone of any nutritional approach to achieving better health and combating disease, there are several reasons why supplements may be useful even for those who eat healthily.

NUTRITIONAL DEFICIENCIES

Scientific studies have shown that nutritional deficiencies are surprisingly common, even in the Western world where food is often plentiful and varied. Modern-day deficiencies are undoubtedly related to food type and quality. Many of the foods available in the average supermarket are relatively high in fat, sugar, and salt, yet low in health-giving elements such as fiber, vitamins, and minerals. Refined and processed foods are often lacking in essential nutrients. For example, in turning wholegrain flour into white flour, 95 percent of the fiber, 60 percent of the calcium, 85 percent of the magnesium, and 78 percent of the zinc are lost. Even fresh fruits and vegetables may be worryingly low in nutrients as a result of poor soil, intensive growing methods, prolonged storage and transportation time, and the use of herbicides and pesticides. Fresh produce is often picked before it is ripe, leading to reduced nutrient content.

WHY USE SUPPLEMENTS?

There is a wealth of evidence linking nutritional deficiencies with a wide range of illnesses including chronic fatigue syndrome, heart disease, and cancer. In some cases the doses of a nutrient needed to achieve the desired health benefit cannot be realistically obtained from the diet. For instance, studies demonstrate that 100 IU of vitamin E a day can reduce the risk of heart disease by 40 percent. It is virtually impossible to obtain this quantity of the vitamin through diet.

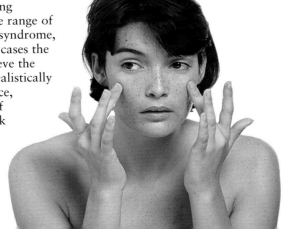

MORE THAN PREVENTING DEFICIENCY

The amount of nutrients needed to prevent, reverse, or treat certain medical conditions is often in excess of the recommended daily allowances (RDAs) of those nutrients. The RDAs are guidelines to the quantities of nutrients that should be taken daily to prevent deficiencies in them. A wealth of scientific research exists which shows that the "optimal" level for certain nutrients is much higher than their current RDAs. For instance, 40 or 60 mg of vitamin C may be enough to prevent scurvy, but is probably not enough to boost immune function and reduce the risk of cancer and heart disease. Furthermore, the RDA does not take account of individual variations in people's needs. It assumes, for instance, that an 18-year-old girl has the same nutritional requirements as an 80-year-old man, and fails to take into consideration lifestyle and environmental factors.

HOW THIS BOOK CAN HELP

This book is intended as a guide to the nutritional approaches and supplements that may benefit a number of conditions. You will find information about the factors that are thought to underlie that condition, as well as the dietary changes that may help prevent or improve it. Guidance is given on the major nutrients that are found to be of benefit. Nutritional supplements are generally to be found in pharmacies and health food stores, and they are also available from reputable mail order companies. For most conditions, several agents are listed. Often, however, it is not necessary to take them all to get benefit – taking one or two can be enough to make a real difference. For more specific guidance, particularly where the condition is a potentially serious one, it is advisable to seek the advice of a qualified professional, such as a nutritionist, naturopath, or herbalist. Many family physicians are also sympathetic to these approaches, and you should discuss any supplements you are taking with your doctor for any condition for which you are also receiving medical care.

MAJOR VITAMINS, MINERALS, AND OTHER NUTRIENTS

The tables on the following pages summarize the actions and benefits of the most commonly used nutritional agents. Where relevant, information is also given on any possible hazards. For dosage, consult the section dealing with the condition being treated.

VITAMINS

Vitamin A

Actions: Helps in the reproduction and development of the body's cells. Helps immune function. Necessary for the production of bone, protein, and growth hormone. Helps maintain the health of the skin and intestinal lining. Has potent antioxidant activity.

Uses: Cervical abnormalities, acne, heavy periods, macular degeneration, cataracts, reduced immune function, peptic ulcers, night blindness.

Cautions: Higher doses should only be used for limited periods of time or they may cause liver damage. Doses of more than 10,000 IU a day should be avoided if you are pregnant or planning pregnancy. People with kidney stones or a history of this condition should seek medical advice before taking vitamin A supplements.

Vitamin B-complex

Actions: B-complex supplements usually contain 10–50 mg of vitamins B_1, B_2, B_3, B_5, B_6, PABA, choline, and inositol and 10–50 mcg of B_{12}, folic acid, and biotin. For details of individual B vitamins, see below.

Cautions: If you are taking the drug levodopa, seek medical advice before taking a B-complex supplement. Prolonged use of isolated B vitamins at high levels may induce a deficiency in some of the other B vitamins. For this reason, it is generally recommended that B vitamins are taken as a complex.

Vitamin B₁ (thiamin)

Actions: Necessary for processing carbohydrates, fats, and protein in the diet, and for the production of the ATP (the basic unit of energy in the body). Important for nerve function.

Uses: Pregnancy.

Cautions: Doses of 75 mg a day should be taken only on medical advice in people with diabetes.

Vitamin B₂ (riboflavin)

Actions: Necessary for the processing of amino acids and fats in the body. Helps in the conversion of carbohydrates into energy.

Uses: Cataracts, athletic performance.

Cautions: Colors urine dark yellow. This has no known adverse effect.

VITAMINS (continued)

Vitamin B3 (niacin, niacinamide)

Actions: Necessary for the release of energy from carbohydrates. Has role to play in the regulation of cholesterol in the blood. Necessary for alcohol processing.

Uses: Pregnancy, cataract, high blood cholesterol.

Cautions: Niacin can cause flushing, headache, and stomachache in doses as low as 50 mg a day. Niacinamide in doses of 100 mg or more a day may aggravate stomach ulcers, glaucoma, and diabetes. 1,000 mg a day or more may impair liver function.

Vitamin B5 (pantothenic acid)

Actions: Involved in energy production in the body. Essential for the processing and transporting of fats. Has a role to play in maintaining the health of the adrenal glands. Needed for the manufacture of the nerve transmitter acetylcholine.

Uses: Athletic performance, rheumatoid arthritis.

Vitamin B6 (pyridoxine)

Actions: Important role in the processing of amino acids.

Uses: Acne, carpal tunnel syndrome, kidney stones, premenstrual syndrome, asthma.

Cautions: Very high doses may cause numbness and tingling in the hands and feet. In pregnancy, doses of over 30 mg a day should be used only under medical supervision.

Vitamin B12 (cobalamin)

Actions: Needed for normal nerve activity. Necessary for DNA replication. Important for the formation of red blood cells.

Uses: Anaemia (pernicious), heart disease.

Cautions: High levels (1,000 mcg or more a day) should be avoided in pregnancy and in children under the age of 12.

Vitamin C

Actions: Needed for the formation of bone, skin, cartilage, tendon, muscle, and blood vessels. Immune-enhancing properties and antioxidant properties. A natural antihistamine. Enhances wound healing.

Uses: Cervical abnormalities, asthma, heart disease, cataracts, colds and flu, eczema, hay fever, male infertility, macular degeneration, glaucoma.

Cautions: May deplete the body of copper. Doses of over 1,000 mg daily are not advised for women taking oral contraceptives. High intake can lead to diarrhea and stomach cramps.

Vitamin D

Actions: Increases absorption of calcium from food. Reduces loss of calcium from the body. Necessary for healthy bones and teeth. May help reduce the risk of cancer.

Uses: Osteoporosis, psoriasis.

Cautions: High doses (more than 1,000 IU a day) can lead to headaches, weight loss, kidney stones, and other complications in the long term.

Vitamin E

Actions: Powerful antioxidant. Protects cholesterol from damage and reduces risk of heart disease. Has natural blood-thinning properties.

Uses: Cervical abnormalities, heart disease, cataracts, macular degeneration, menopause, fibrocystic breast disease.

Cautions: People with high blood pressure should avoid doses in excess of 100 IU a day. If you are taking anticoagulant drugs such as warfarin or heparin, avoid vitamin E except under medical supervision.

Vitamin K

Actions: Important for bone formation and blood clotting. Helps in calcium transport around body.

Uses: Osteoporosis, morning sickness.

Cautions: Those taking anticoagulant drugs such as warfarin or heparin should avoid vitamin K except under medical supervision.

MINERALS

Boron

Actions: Increases the absorption of calcium, magnesium, and phosphorus.

Uses: Osteoporosis, arthritis.

Cautions: May increase estrogen levels in the body.

Calcium

Actions: Necessary for healthy bones and teeth and for the nervous system. Required for normal muscle contraction.

Uses: High blood pressure, osteoporosis, pregnancy, kidney stones.

Cautions: Calcium supplementation should be avoided if you have sarcoidosis, hyperparathyroidism, or chronic kidney disease.

MINERALS (continued)

Chromium

Actions: Has an essential role in the maintenance of blood sugar levels and in maintaining healthy levels of cholesterol in the blood.
Uses: Diabetes, hypoglycemia, obesity, high blood cholesterol.
Cautions: Do not take if you are pregnant. Take only on medical advice for diabetes.

Copper

Actions: Necessary for the absorption and utilization of iron. It is involved in the formation of ATP (the basic unit of energy in the body) and collagen.
Uses: Osteoporosis.
Cautions: Copper supplements should not be taken by those with Wilson's disease.

Iodine

Actions: Necessary for the manufacture of thyroid hormones.
Uses: Thyroid disease.

Iron

Actions: Necessary for the production of hemoglobin in red blood cells. Involved in the production of ATP (the basic unit of energy in the body).
Uses: Athletic performance, anemia, heavy periods.
Cautions: May be dangerous in overdose. May cause constipation. Avoid if you have hemochromatosis, hemosiderosis, polycythemia, thallasemia, or sickle-cell anemia.

Magnesium

Actions: Necessary for bone formation and new cell manufacture. Has a muscle-relaxing effect. Activates some B vitamins. Is involved in the production of ATP (the basic unit of energy in the body). Important for insulin secretion and function.
Uses: Asthma, athletic performance, high blood pressure, kidney stones, headaches (including migraine), osteoporosis, premenstrual syndrome, abnormal heart rhythms.
Cautions: May cause diarrhea. Avoid if you have a history of kidney disease.

Potassium

Actions: Helps regulate water balance and blood pressure. Necessary for carbohydrate and protein metabolism. Important for nerve and muscle function.
Uses: High blood pressure, kidney stones, cramp.
Cautions: May cause stomach irritation. Should not be used if you have kidney disease or are taking potassium-sparing diuretics ("water pills").

Selenium

Actions: Activates an enzyme called glutathione peroxidase which has antioxidant activity. Has an anticancer role in the body.

Uses: Cancer prevention, macular degeneration, cervical abnormalities.

Cautions: Levels above 200 mcg a day should be taken only on medical advice.

Zinc

Actions: Helps maintain fertility and vision. Important in wound healing and in the synthesis of protein in the body. Enhances immune function. Has a role in cell division.

Uses: Acne, anorexia nervosa, prostate disease, colds and flu, male infertility, macular degeneration, night blindness, peptic ulcers, wound healing.

Cautions: Doses in excess of 300 mg a day may impair the immune response.

OTHER NUTRIENTS

Acidophilus

Actions: Enhances digestion, improves the health of the intestinal lining, and increases resistance to digestive-tract infections.

Uses: Irritable bowel syndrome, yeast, cystitis.

Biotin

Actions: Necessary for the metabolism of carbohydrates, protein, and fat.

Uses: Brittle nails, poor hair growth.

Choline

Actions: Vitaminlike substance often included in B-complex supplements. Important for nerve function. Helps to remove fat from the liver.

Uses: Gallbladder disease.

Coenzyme Q10 (Co-Q10, ubiquinone)

Actions: Has potent antioxidant activity in the body. Is essential for the generation of ATP (the body's basic unit of energy).

Uses: Angina, heart failure, gum disease, fatigue, athletic performance.

Cautions: People taking Coenzyme Q10 for heart failure should not discontinue it abruptly as this may worsen their condition.

Fish oil

Actions: Rich in the essential fats EPA (eicosapentaenoic acid) and DHA (docosahexanoic acid), fish oil helps to reduce triglycerides (a type of fat) in the blood and reduce blood clotting. EPA and DHA also have anti-inflammatory activity.

Uses: Eczema, high cholesterol and triglyceride levels, rheumatoid arthritis, osteoarthritis, high blood pressure, psoriasis.

OTHER NUTRIENTS (continued)

Folic acid

Actions: Necessary for the formation of red cells in the blood. Necessary for the synthesis of DNA, which is important for normal cell replication. Has a role in preventing neural-tube defects (e.g. spina bifida) in the developing fetus.

Uses: Anemia, cervical abnormalities, heart disease, pregnancy.

Cautions: High doses may mask symptoms of anemia caused by B_{12} deficiency. High doses (1,000 mcg or more a day) should be avoided by people taking methotrexate.

Gamma linolenic acid

Actions: The active ingredient in evening primrose oil, starflower oil, borage oil, and blackcurrant seed oil. Has anti-inflammatory and blood thinning properties.

Uses: Dry skin, dry eyes, fibrocystic breast disease, eczema, premenstrual syndrome.

Glucosamine sulfate

Actions: The main building block in the manufacture of cartilage, tendon, and ligament tissues.

Uses: Osteoarthritis.

Inositol

Actions: Important for the formation of cell membranes. Has a role in nerve transmission. Assists in the transportation of fat in the body.

Uses: Depression.

Linseed oil

Actions: Rich in two essential fats – linoleic acid and alpha linolenic acid (ALA).

Uses: Prostate disease.

Lutein

Actions: An antioxidant related to vitamin A and betacarotene.

Uses: Cataracts, macular degeneration.

Lycopene

Actions: Related to betacarotene, lycopene has antioxidant effects in the body.

Uses: Cancer risk reduction.

Lysine

Actions: An essential amino acid. Interferes with the replication of the herpes virus.

Uses: Herpes infections (cold sores and genital herpes).

Quercetin

Actions: Antihistamine and anti-inflammatory effects in the body.

Uses: Hay fever, asthma.

Everyday Health

EVERYDAY HEALTH

Many of us suffer from complaints and symptoms which may not be serious enough to take us to see our doctor but, nevertheless, can be troublesome and worrying. Conditions such as fatigue, headaches, and insomnia are common problems, the causes of which are often poorly understood in conventional medical terms. This chapter covers some of the common everyday symptoms we may experience and offers explanations for their causes, together with advice on dietary changes and nutritional supplements that may help. This chapter also offers alternative strategies for the treatment of medical conditions such as peptic ulcers and depression that may be of benefit for anyone who has found conventional treatment to be ineffective, or who would prefer a more natural solution to their problem.

SUPPLEMENTS AT ALL AGES

The value of nutritional supplements to maintain health and treat disease is well proven. Nutrients have an impact on our well-being from the time we are conceived until old age. However, the precise nutrients that are important for optimum health change as we develop and mature. While a healthy diet coupled with a good quality multivitamin and mineral preparation may help ensure that the bulk of our dietary needs are met, special emphasis on certain nutrients may be appropriate at various stages in our life.

USEFUL SUPPLEMENTS

Supplement	Action	Dose
Children		
Multivitamin and mineral preparation	An over-reliance on highly refined foods which can be high in fat, sugar, and artificial additives and low in health-giving elements such as fiber, vitamins, and minerals has meant that the nutritional quality of children's diets has been declining for some time. Low levels of nutrients in the diet may ultimately lead to a variety of problems including growth retardation, problems with behavior and concentration, and learning difficulties. Giving a child a multivitamin and mineral preparation specifically designed for children is likely to prevent potential nutritional deficiencies and optimize health in the longer term.	Follow the instructions on the label
Teenagers		
Calcium	Calcium is important to maintain healthy bone growth. Studies show that girls who consume more calcium have better bone development.	500 mg a day
Zinc	Zinc is an important mineral for the development of the reproductive organs, and there is an increased need for this mineral during the teenage years. Zinc can also help combat acne, which is a common problem at this time.	15 mg a day

Supplement	Action	Dose
20s and 30s		
Iron	Women suffering from heavy periods can become iron deficient, which may lead to anemia. But iron should be supplemented only once a diagnosis of iron deficiency has been established by a doctor.	50–100 mg of iron a day as required
Folic acid	Low levels of folic acid are linked to an increased risk of having a child with spina bifida. Women planning pregnancy should take supplements for three months before conception and during the first three months of pregnancy.	400 mcg a day
Antioxidant formulation	Antioxidants such as vitamins A, C, and E and the mineral selenium combat the damaging effects of stress, pollution, alcohol, and a diet high in animal fat. Antioxidant nutrients also help in the production of healthy sperm.	Follow the instructions on the label
Zinc	An important nutrient for men as it has an essential role to play in sperm formation.	30 mg a day
40s and 50s		
Calcium	Important for women who may be at risk of osteoporosis.	1000 mg a day
Magnesium	Another essential bone-building mineral.	500 mg a day
Vitamin E	Vitamin E supplementation can lead to a 40 percent reduction of risk from heart disease.	200 IU a day
Selenium	Supplementation with this antioxidant may dramatically reduce the risk of developing cancer.	200 mcg a day

60s and beyond
Continue to take calcium, magnesium, vitamin E, and selenium as above plus:

Ginkgo biloba	This herb improves circulation, combating cold hands and feet, a common problem in older people. Improved blood supply to the brain can also improve memory and mental function.	40 mg of standardized extract three times a day

FATIGUE

O f all the everyday complaints from which people suffer, fatigue and lack of vitality are perhaps the most common. Lack of energy can be due to a wide variety of factors including anemia, an under-active thyroid gland, and diabetes. Anyone suffering from persistent fatigue should see their doctor so that appropriate tests can be performed.

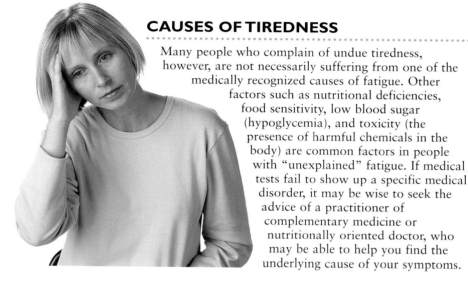

CAUSES OF TIREDNESS

Many people who complain of undue tiredness, however, are not necessarily suffering from one of the medically recognized causes of fatigue. Other factors such as nutritional deficiencies, food sensitivity, low blood sugar (hypoglycemia), and toxicity (the presence of harmful chemicals in the body) are common factors in people with "unexplained" fatigue. If medical tests fail to show up a specific medical disorder, it may be wise to seek the advice of a practitioner of complementary medicine or nutritionally oriented doctor, who may be able to help you find the underlying cause of your symptoms.

DIET ESSENTIALS

Whatever the cause of your fatigue, a healthy diet is essential for overcoming it. The food we eat provides the fuel on which our body runs, and if the fuel is not of the right type, the body cannot function efficiently. As a general rule, the diet should be based around nutritious foods that readily supply energy to the body, including fresh fruits, vegetables, wholegrain starches, such as whole-wheat bread and brown rice, beans, and legumes. Avoid foodstuffs that tend to sap the body of energy. These include red meat, dairy products, processed foods, fried foods, foods containing artificial additives, sugar, caffeine, and alcohol.

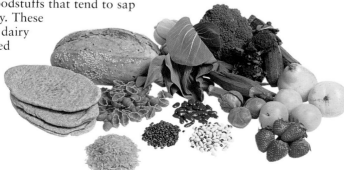

USEFUL SUPPLEMENTS

The following supplements may help to revive flagging energy levels:

Supplement	Action	Dose
B-complex	The B-complex vitamins play an essential role in the reactions that unlock energy from food. Many people find that supplementing with additional quantities of B vitamins (particularly vitamins B_2, B_5, and B_6) can help boost their energy levels.	B-complex supplement containing 25–50 mg of vitamins B_1–B_6 each day
Coenzyme Q10	The processes that generate energy from food take place inside each cell in minute powerhouses called the mitochondria. Here, energy in food is converted into molecules of a substance called ATP, which the body then uses to generate energy. Coenzyme Q10 (also known as Co-Q10 and ubiquinone) is a key catalyst in the process that generates ATP. Supplementing with Coenzyme Q10 has been found to improve energy levels and increase work capacity.	30–50 mg three times a day
Chromium	A great number of people who complain of unexplained tiredness tend to run a blood sugar level lower than it should be – a condition known as hypoglycemia. Other common symptoms of this condition include food cravings, irritability, and poor concentration. Chromium supplements have been shown to help maintain blood sugar levels in the body.	200–400 mcg a day. Avoid in pregnancy
Siberian ginseng	Used in Chinese medicine as a general tonic and energy booster, Siberian ginseng's effects are quite similar to those of caffeine, and studies have shown it can sharpen the mind as well as improve physical energy. However, Siberian ginseng does not tend to cause the energy drop that is a characteristic after-effect of caffeinated products. Use Siberian ginseng on a cyclical basis with treatment periods of six to eight weeks interspersed with breaks lasting two weeks. Some people experience mild diarrhea and insomnia.	300–400 mg of solid concentrated standardized extract a day

HEADACHES AND MIGRAINE

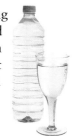

Headaches can be caused by a variety of factors, including eyestrain, tension, the inhalation of toxic fumes, and certain dietary factors. On a dietary level, a very common cause of headache is dehydration. If you suffer from frequent headaches, make sure you drink at least 2¹/₂ pints of filtered or spring water each day.

CAFFEINE AND HEADACHES

Another common cause of headaches is caffeine withdrawal. Anyone used to drinking caffeinated tea, coffee, or soft drinks on a regular basis will normally find that they experience a headache if they abstain for a day or two. The headaches that some people experience at the weekend can sometimes be due to caffeine withdrawal. This problem can be overcome by switching to decaffeinated drinks or naturally caffeine-free beverages such as herb and fruit teas.

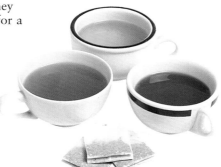

MIGRAINE AND ITS TRIGGERS

Migraine is a common condition, affecting one in ten of the adult population. Migraine headaches tend to be more severe than run-of-the-mill headaches and tend to affect only one side of the head. An attack may sometimes be preceded by some form of visual disturbance such as flashing lights or partial blindness. Attacks tend to last from two hours to two days. Migraine headaches may be triggered by stress, but there is increasing evidence that certain foods are known to trigger migraine. Sometimes referred to as "the five Cs," these are: chocolate, cheese, claret (and other red wines), coffee, and citrus fruits. If you are susceptible to migraines, try to avoid these foods along with certain others that also seem to be associated with migraine such as aged, cured, pickled, soured, yeasty, or fermented foods.

STABILIZING BLOOD SUGAR

Migraine can sometimes be triggered if the level of sugar in the bloodstream gets too low (hypoglycemia). To maintain a stable level of blood sugar, keep your diet based around fresh fruits and vegetables, meat, fish, and wholegrain starches like whole-wheat bread, whole-wheat pasta, and brown rice. All these foods give a sustained release of sugar into the bloodstream that helps keep the blood sugar from dropping too low. Conversely try to avoid foods that promote a rapid rise in blood sugar, which tends to be followed by a sudden drop in the level of sugar in the blood. Foods that contain a high proportion of sugar or refined carbohydrates are most likely to have this effect. It is important to eat regularly, so don't skip meals. Many people need to eat more frequently than the standard three meals a day, so allow yourself a healthy snack if you feel yourself getting over-hungry.

USEFUL SUPPLEMENTS		
Supplement	**Action**	**Dose**
Magnesium	Headaches can be associated with magnesium deficiency. Supplementing with this mineral may help a significant proportion of sufferers.	250 mg twice a day
If headaches or migraines can be triggered by a skipped meal		
Chromium	Chromium helps to stabilize blood sugar levels and may help to prevent headaches caused by low blood sugar. Avoid in pregnancy.	200 mcg twice a day
B-complex	These nutrients help to stabilize blood sugar and may therefore reduce the frequency and severity of headaches and migraine.	25–50 mg a day
For migraine		
Feverfew	In tests, this herb has been found to reduce the frequency, severity, and duration of migraine attacks. Avoid in children under two, in pregnancy, and during breastfeeding.	250 mg a day of feverfew's active ingredient parthenolide

SLEEPING PROBLEMS

Insomnia is a common problem that isn't always the result of stress or an overactive mind, and may well be related to nutritional factors. For instance, one common cause of sleeplessness is caffeine, due to its powerful stimulant effects in the body. Another frequent sleep disrupter is alcohol. Although it may initially have a calming effect, alcohol actually interferes with deep sleep. Avoiding both caffeine and alcohol in the afternoon and evening may well help to improve the quantity and quality of your sleep.

STIMULATING AND SEDATING FOODS

It's not just what you drink, but also what you eat, that may affect your sleep. Protein-rich foods tend to increase mental alertness and are therefore best avoided if you have trouble dropping off to sleep. The foods to minimize or avoid altogether at supper include meat, fish, and cheese. An evening meal based around carbohydrates, such as brown rice or whole-wheat pasta, has a more calming effect on the brain and can actually aid sleep.

NIGHTTIME WAKEFULNESS

While some people have difficulty dropping off to sleep, others have the problem of waking in the middle of the night. During sleep, the body continues to regulate important internal processes. One essential task the body has during the night is to keep the level of sugar in the bloodstream constant. If the blood sugar level drops, the body secretes certain hormones to correct this. These hormones also tend to increase wakefulness. The secret to ensuring a good night's sleep for many individuals is to maintain a stable level of blood sugar throughout the night.

ELECTROMAGNETIC POLLUTION

People who have a lot of electronic gadgetry in the bedroom often find sleep difficult. The electromagnetic energy that these devices emit, even when switched off, can disrupt sleep patterns. Remove such equipment from your bedroom to improve your quality of sleep. A battery-operated alarm clock is a good alternative to an electric clock radio.

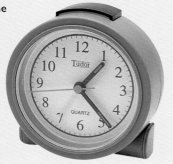

PREVENTING LOW BLOOD SUGAR AT NIGHT

Avoid foods and drinks – particularly at your evening meal – that release sugar quickly into the bloodstream such as candy, dessert, white bread, white rice, pasta, and potatoes. There is a tendency for the body to overcompensate for the rapid rise in blood sugar these foods produce. This leads to low blood sugar later on. If you eat carbohydrates late at night, it is important that they are in their unrefined (whole) form. They then release sugar slowly into the bloodstream, helping to maintain adequate blood sugar levels throughout the night. Having a light snack before bedtime can also help keep sugar levels up during the night.

■ A couple of rye crackers with a nonsweet topping is a good choice.

■ Lettuce is thought to have sedative properties, so a whole-wheat salad sandwich could also be a soothing late-night snack.

■ Bananas are also supposed to be sleep-inducing. A bowl of unsweetened granola with banana could therefore be another good choice.

USEFUL SUPPLEMENTS

Supplement	Action	Dose
Magnesium	Magnesium has a calming effect on the brain and can therefore aid sleep.	500 mg with your evening meal
Passiflora and valerian	Herbal extracts of the plants passiflora (passion flower) and valerian are renowned for their sleep-inducing and sedative properties. Take an hour before bedtime. Avoid alcohol.	Follow the instructions on the label
Chromium	Chromium helps the body regulate blood sugar levels and may therefore help prevent waking in the night. Avoid in pregnancy.	200–400 mcg with your evening meal

ANXIETY AND DEPRESSION

Although anxiety is often thought of as a purely psychological condition, the stress it puts on the body is associated with a wide range of physical conditions. Anxiety can suppress the function of the immune system, making us more prone to infections such as colds or flu. Stress is also thought to be a contributing factor in some of the major killers, including heart disease and cancer.

WHAT IS ANXIETY?

Heightened emotions, feeings of restlessness, and feeling constantly on edge are the hallmark of anxiety. When you are anxious, you find it hard to concentrate and may suffer from physical symptoms such as palpitations, feelings of tightness in the chest, headaches, and stomach cramps. What is happening is that the body is releasing adrenalin, a hormone that primes the body for action, in response to a perceived threat. Some of the symptoms of anxiety can have a physical cause, so it is important to seek an expert medical diagnosis.

WHAT IS DEPRESSION?

Depression is normally associated with low mood and feelings of unhappiness. While it is normal for us to have feelings of unhappiness from time to time in response to adverse life events such as marital or work problems, true depression is normally accompanied by other symptoms, such as disturbed sleep, low self-esteem, and poor appetite. The causes of depression are complex and not fully understood, but changes in the chemical balance in the brain may be responsible.

Warning

Anyone who feels severely depressed and/or has contemplated suicide should seek immediate help from a doctor or mental health care professional.

UPSETTING THE CHEMICAL BALANCE

The brain is a very finely tuned organ, and its balance can be quite easily upset by certain foods or nutritional deficiencies. Caffeine and sugar are commonly associated with depression, and eliminating them from the diet can help lift the mood in as little as a week. Caffeine has potent stimulatory effects on both the mind and body, and can trigger or worsen anxiety and such associated symptoms as sleeplessness and palpitations. Alcohol is a common cause of depression, and cutting it out for a month may well help improve your mood.

USEFUL SUPPLEMENTS

Supplement	Action	Dose
ANXIETY		
B-complex	B vitamins have a very important role to play in the body as an antidote to stress and anxiety. Take a supplement that contains the major B vitamins – B_1, B_2, B_3, B_5, and B_6.	25–50 mg a day
Siberian ginseng	Ginseng has been used for thousands of years as a tonic. It appears that ginseng helps the body withstand stress of all kinds. It is generally recommended that ginseng be used on a cyclical basis with treatment periods of six to eight weeks interspersed with breaks of two weeks. Some people experience mild diarrhea and insomnia. Siberian ginseng is thought of as a relatively mild form of ginseng and tends to cause fewer problems with insomnia than other types.	300–400 mg of solid concentrated standardized extract a day
Kava kava	This herb has been found to be effective in the treatment of nervous anxiety and restlessness. It is a natural tranquilizer and can promote a feeling of general well-being.	Follow the instructions on the label
DEPRESSION		
Vitamin C	Deficiency of vitamin C seems to be a factor in some cases of depression. Women taking oral contraceptives should take a maximum daily dose of no more than 1000 mg.	500 mg three times a day
Hypericum perforatum (St. John's wort)	Several trials looking at the properties of this herb show that it can be as effective as conventional antidepressants in mild and moderate depression, but has few, if any, side effects. Discuss with your doctor if you are taking prescribed antidepressants. Avoid during pregnancy and breastfeeding.	300 mcg of standardized hypericin extract three times a day

ACID REFLUX AND ULCERS

When we swallow, food passes down a tube called the esophagus into the stomach. Just before it opens into the stomach, the esophagus passes through a sheet of muscle called the diaphragm. Sometimes, part of the stomach is pulled up through the diaphragm – a condition known as hiatus hernia. This allows stomach acid to escape into the esophagus – acid reflux. Symptoms include heartburn and digestive discomfort. Abdominal pain associated with eating may also be caused by ulcers in the lining of the stomach or duodenum (the tube leading from the stomach).

CHANGING YOUR EATING HABITS

Nutritional therapy can often control the symptoms of acid reflux. You need to avoid large meals. This is especially true at night, because lying down makes it much more likely that acid will escape from the stomach. Eat your evening meal at least three hours before going to bed to allow most of the food you have eaten to pass out of the stomach before you retire. Propping yourself up in bed with some pillows may also help.

EASING THE SYMPTOMS

Anything you can do to ease digestion can also help to reduce the symptoms of a hiatus hernia. Chew your food very thoroughly and avoid drinking with meals. Adopting the principles of food combining – separating protein and starch at each meal – is also usually effective in combating symptoms.

FOOD COMBINING GROUPS

Protein	Neutral	Starch
Any protein can be eaten with any neutral food		
Meats	All green and	Bread
Fish	root vegetables	Rice
Shellfish	except potatoes	Pasta
Dairy products	Salad vegetables	Cereal
Soybeans and	Nuts and seeds	Potatoes
bean curd	Cream	Flour-based foods
	Butter	Cookies
	Vegetable oils	Dried fruits
		Bananas
		Mangoes
		Sugar and honey

Any starch can be eaten with any neutral food

PEPTIC ULCERS

Indigestion may sometimes be caused by an ulcer in the stomach or first part of the small intestine, called the duodenum. The lining of the gut is shielded from potentially damaging digestive secretions by a coating of protective mucus. Sometimes, this protective mechanism breaks down, leading to the development of a raw area or ulcer in the wall of the intestine. Many ulcers seem to be caused by a bacterium known as Helicobacter pylori, and the possibility of this should be discussed with your doctor.

ULCER-HEALING THROUGH DIET

Dietary changes and certain nutritional supplements may promote ulcer healing and help prevent a recurrence of the problem. Sugar, alcohol, coffee, and tea should all be avoided, because all these foodstuffs seem to increase the risk of developing an ulcer or slow down its healing. A high-fiber diet seems to prevent recurrence of ulcers once they have healed, so make sure you eat plenty of fiber-rich foods such as oats, brown rice, fruits, and vegetables. Cabbage juice is very effective in healing ulcers. You will need a juicer to make this, but relief from discomfort may occur within days. Drink a pint of cabbage juice gradually throughout the day. Dilute with water if you find the taste too strong.

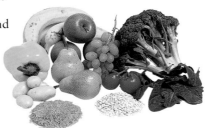

USEFUL SUPPLEMENTS

Supplement	Action	Dose
Vitamin A	Vitamin A can be beneficial in healing ulcers because it enhances tissue healing. Seek medical advice if you have a history of kidney stones. Do not take more than 10,000 IU a day if you are pregnant or planning pregnancy.	10,000 IU a day (women); 25,000 IU a day (men)
Zinc	Zinc promotes tissue healing.	30 mg a day
Deglycyrrhizin-ated licorice (DGL)	This compound has been shown to be about as effective as conventional drugs in healing ulcers. Take doses 15 minutes before meals and 1–2 hours before bedtime.	250–500 mg
Slippery elm	This has a general soothing and healing effect on the lining of the stomach.	800–1000 mg 3–4 times a day

CONSTIPATION

The main function of the large bowel is to eliminate waste from the body. However, many individuals in the Western world experience problems with constipation, where the stool is difficult to pass, or bowel movements are too infrequent for comfort. Constipation can increase the risk of certain bowel conditions such as diverticular disease and cancer of the colon. Constipation also increases the likelihood of hemorrhoids (piles), dilated veins around the anus which cause discomfort and pain, and may bleed. Also, if waste products are not eliminated efficiently from the body, toxicity can build up leading to problems such as headaches, fatigue, and poor skin.

FIBER AND FLUID

One essential ingredient for healthy bowel function is fiber. Many people turn to high-bran breakfast cereals as a means of increasing their fiber intake. The fiber in these cereals is quite hard and scratchy and may irritate the delicate lining of the gut. The fiber found in oats, fresh fruits, and vegetables is generally kinder to the gut, and the consumption of these foods should be increased. Apart from fiber, the other essential ingredient for bowel regularity is water. Without enough water, the stool can become quite dry, and this may cause it to become stuck, a bit like a cork in the neck of a wine bottle. If you do suffer from constipation, make sure you drink 2$^1/_2$–3$^1/_2$ pints of filtered or spring water each day.

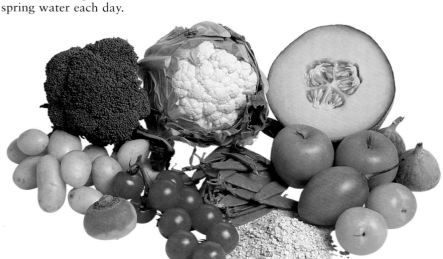

THE NEED FOR EXERCISE

Constipation can also be related to a sedentary lifestyle. The large bowel moves waste material along it using a rhythmical contraction known as peristalsis. Exercises such as brisk walking, jogging, and aerobics may help stimulate peristalsis and are well known to assist the large bowel's efficient functioning. Aim at taking about 30 minutes of exercise, at least every other day. Choose a form of exercise to suit your fitness level. If you have been leading a sedentary life, check with your doctor first.

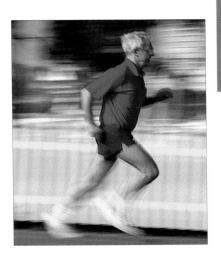

USEFUL SUPPLEMENTS

Supplement	Action	Dose
Linseeds	An effective and convenient way to increase your fiber intake is to add linseeds to your diet. These small golden seeds can really help to improve bowel regularity. Take either sprinkled on cereal or with water.	One tablespoon a day
Psyllium	Psyllium powder is an alternative to linseeds. Add to a glass of water and drink. Follow this with another two glasses of water.	About 2 teaspoons a day
Vitamin C	In high doses, vitamin C can be effective in remedying constipation. The most economical way to take large doses of vitamin C is as a powder. Women taking oral contraceptives should take a maximum daily dose of 1000 mg.	1–3 grams of vitamin C in divided doses throughout the day
Magnesium	Magnesium can improve the function of the muscles in the large bowel and may help to ease constipation.	200 mg once or twice a day

IRRITABLE BOWEL

Irritable bowel syndrome (IBS) is a common digestive problem, typical symptoms of which are bloating, excessive flatulence, abdominal discomfort, and constipation and/or loose bowels. Anyone with these symptoms should consult his or her doctor so that potentially serious conditions can be ruled out.

FOODS TO AVOID

Many everyday foods seem to be potential causes of irritable bowel syndrome. Cheese and wheat are common culprits. You may notice a marked improvement in symptoms if you eliminate cheese, bread, pasta, cookies, cakes, and wheat-based cereals and crackers from your diet. Other foods to avoid include yeast-containing foods such as stock cubes and yeast extract, dried fruits, and high sugar foods.

FOODS THAT HELP

Soybean cheese and potatoes, rice, rice cakes, rye crackers, and oat-based cereals, such as porridge, are useful substitutes for the wheat and cheese products that are often responsible for provoking symptoms of irritable bowel syndrome. It is also helpful to eat a high-fiber diet. However, avoid eating too much cereal fiber, such as bran. The fiber present in fruits, vegetables, and legumes is much gentler on the bowel. Drink plenty of fluids, preferably in the form of plain water or herb teas such as peppermint or fennel. Caffeine-containing and high-sugar drinks can make symptoms worse.

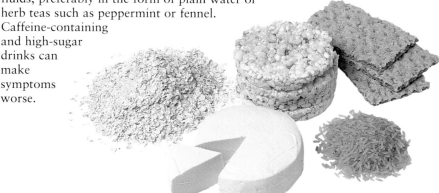

THE BACTERIA OF THE GUT

Apart from food sensitivity, the other major underlying cause of irritable bowel syndrome is an imbalance in the organisms that live in the gut – also known as gut dysbiosis. The intestinal tract normally contains about 3–4¹/₂ pounds of bacteria which have an important part to play in digestion and in keeping the lining of the gut healthy.

However, in certain circumstances significant quantities of healthy gut bacteria can be lost, allowing potentially harmful organisms such as yeast to overgrow. This imbalance in the population of organisms in the gut may lead to the symptoms of irritable bowel syndrome.

CAUSES OF GUT DYSBIOSIS

Common factors that may lead to the development of gut dysbiosis include the taking of antibiotics, long-term use of the oral contraceptive pill, prolonged stress, and a diet high in sugar and refined carbohydrates, such as white bread and pasta. Eating live yogurt on a daily basis is one of the simplest ways of restoring and maintaining a healthy population of bacteria in the gut. For more details about how to restore better balance to the gut, read the section on yeast on pages 104–5.

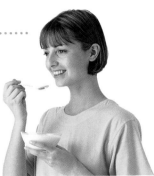

USEFUL SUPPLEMENTS

Supplement	Action	Dose
Acidophilus	Acidophilus is one of the most important species of healthy bacteria in the gut. Taking it in supplement form can really help to restore better balance to the intestinal ecosystem, which often has a very beneficial effect on the symptoms of IBS. For maximum potency, acidophilus supplements should be kept refrigerated.	1–10 billion live organisms a day
Aloe vera	Extracts of the aloe vera cactus plant have been found to help symptoms in many sufferers of IBS. Aloe vera has many functions in the gut, including healing and antimicrobial properties.	30 ml of gel three times a day
Peppermint oil	Peppermint oil contains substances that can ease spasm in the gut wall.	Follow the instructions on the label

LACTOSE INTOLERANCE

In many cases symptoms of irritable bowel syndrome are triggered by cow's milk. Milk seems to provoke symptoms in many sufferers because of an inability to digest the sugar in milk called lactose. Lactose is normally broken down in the gut before its constituents are absorbed through the intestinal wall into the bloodstream.

QUICK TEST

Buy some lactose from the pharmacist. Mix a tablespoon in some water and drink. If symptoms appear within a few hours, lactose intolerance is likely to be the cause of your problem.

Soy milk and rice milk provide suitable alternatives to cow's milk for those with lactose intolerance.

HOW SYMPTOMS ARE CAUSED

Lactase is an enzyme normally produced in the gut that is responsible for digesting lactose. Some people lack this enzyme, which can give rise to symptoms such as diarrhea, bloating, and flatulence when foods containing lactose are eaten. This condition is called "lactose intolerance." It can be present at birth or can develop in later life, sometimes as a result of a bout of gastroenteritis. Lactase deficiency sometimes corrects itself. People of African and Asian origin are more likely to suffer from permanent lactase deificiency. Try cutting out milk or switching to a lactose-reduced milk to see if this improves your symptoms.

USEFUL SUPPLEMENTS

Supplement	Action	Dose
Lactase	Lactase is the enzyme responsible for digesting lactose in the gut. If there is any suspicion of lactose intolerance, preparations of this enzyme may be used either to treat milk prior to consumption, or as a supplement when you consume milk or milk-containing food.	Follow the instructions on the label

Skin and Eyes

SKIN AND EYES

The health of our skin can have a profound influence on our confidence and how we feel about ourselves. Skin conditions such as acne and psoriasis can impact on many areas of our lives. The conventional medical approach to many skin problems is to treat the skin itself, often with medications that may damage it in the long term. This chapter explains the factors at work in common skin conditions and offers natural strategies to combat them. In addition to skin ailments, this chapter also covers conditions that may affect our sight including cataracts and macular degeneration. Nutritional supplements have been found to be effective in halting and, in some cases, reversing common eye conditions.

2

GENERAL SKIN HEALTH

2

The skin, like every tissue in the body, is constantly renewing itself. The raw materials that the body uses to regenerate skin on an on-going basis come from what we eat and drink. This means that dietary factors have an important role to play in the general health of our skin. While we may invest in creams and lotions for our skin, the real secret to healthy skin is to feed it from within.

FEEDING YOUR SKIN

Anyone who wants to make sure that his or her skin is healthy and glowing should eat a diet rich in the nutrients that have an important part to play in skin health. Key nutrients include zinc, the essential fatty acids, betacarotene, and vitamins C and E. Your diet should therefore be rich in fresh fruits and vegetables (betacarotene, and vitamins C and E), seafood and seeds (zinc), oily fish and extra-virgin olive oil (essential fatty acids). Water is important for skin health, both to keep it moist and also to assist in the removal of toxins through it. Be sure to drink about 2$^1/_2$ pints of filtered or spring water every day.

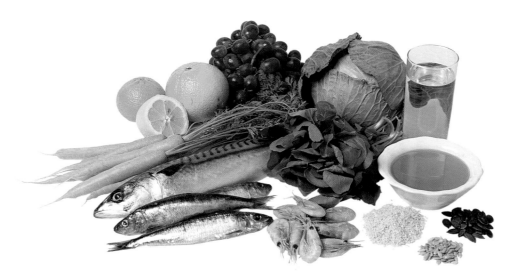

THE CAUSES OF PREMATURE AGING

The effects of aging in the skin are largely caused by damaging destructive substances in the body called "free radicals." These rogue molecules wreak havoc in the skin, damaging the cells and protein structures that make up the substance of the skin. Certain factors stimulate the production of free radicals in the body and therefore speed the aging processes in the skin. These include stress, the consumption of unhealthful (animal) fat, smoking, excessive exposure to the sun's ultraviolet rays, and pollution. These factors should be avoided wherever possible. The effects of free radicals on the skin can also be combated by nutrients known as antioxidants which include betacarotene, vitamins A, C, and E, and the mineral selenium.

2

USEFUL SUPPLEMENTS

Supplement	Action	Dose
Vitamin C	Vitamin C helps to neutralize the effects of free radicals. Vitamin C is also essential for the production of a protein called collagen which provides support for the skin. Women taking oral contraceptives should take a maximum daily dose of no more than 1000 mg.	500 mg three times a day
Vitamin E	Vitamin E, an antioxidant, is known to enhance skin health.	400 IU a day
Betacarotene	Has general skin-feeding properties as well as helping to protect the skin from the effects of the sun's rays.	25,000 IU a day
Zinc	The mineral zinc is important for the general integrity of the skin and is essential for adequate wound healing.	15–45 mg a day
Evening primrose oil or Starflower oil	The essential fats contained in these supplements help keep skin soft, smooth, and velvety.	1 g three times a day 500 mg three times a day

ACNE

Acne is caused by blockages in the glands of the skin responsible for making the skin's protective oil called sebum. In adolescents and young adults the development of acne is often related to hormonal changes. Antibiotics are often prescribed for persistent acne, but while these sometimes improve the condition of the skin, they may also kill many of the healthy bacteria in the gut. In the longer term, this may lead to other problems, such as irritable bowel syndrome (see Irritable Bowel, page 28).

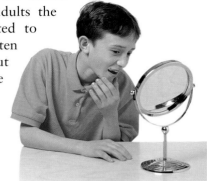

2

DIETARY MEASURES

There is a great deal of controversy over the role of diet in the development of acne. While some sufferers report that dietary changes have little impact on their symptoms, for others such changes produce a big improvement. Acne sufferers tend to consume more animal fat and sugar than individuals with healthy skin, and for this reason, you should cut down on consumption of dairy products, red meat, processed foods, candy, and soft drinks. Base your diet instead on fresh fruits and vegetables, fish, and whole grains such as brown rice and whole-wheat bread. You should also drink 2½–3½ pints of filtered or bottled spring water each day to keep your body well hydrated and free from toxins.

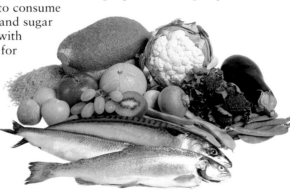

PREMENSTRUAL ACNE

Some women find that their skin condition worsens in the few days prior to their period. Premenstrual acne often responds well to supplementation with vitamin B₆. Take 50 mg 1–2 times a day in the week or so before you expect to start your period.

USEFUL SUPPLEMENTS

Supplement	Action	Dose
Zinc	This mineral can be very effective in reducing spots and acne because it strengthens the immune system and promotes wound healing.	40–60 mg a day for two months, then 15–20 mg a day
Betacarotene	Betacarotene is converted into vitamin A in the body. Both these nutrients have important roles to play in the health of the skin and are known to be effective in the treatment of acne.	25,000– 50,000 IU a day
Vitamin E	Vitamin E has generally beneficial effects on the skin.	400 IU a day
Selenium	Selenium may help in the treatment of skin problems, possibly through its antioxidant and immune-enhancing properties.	200 mcg a day
Acidophilus	If you have taken antibiotics to control acne, it is likely that there will be some element of imbalance of the organisms in the intestinal tract. It is important that healthy gut bacteria is replenished if balance in the ecosystem within the gut is to be restored. Take a good-quality acidophilus supplement for two months.	Follow the instructions on the label
Tea tree oil	Tea tree oil has potent antibacterial properties and may help to control the infection and inflammation that is characteristic of acne.	Apply sparingly twice a day to affected areas

2

ECZEMA

Eczema is characterized by a red, often itchy rash, which may cause the skin to become cracked and sore. Typical body sites affected include the face, hands, inside of the elbows, and the back of the knees. Eczema is caused by inflammation in the outer layers of the skin. Although such inflammation can sometimes be caused by some external irritant such as cleaning fluid or wool, or psychological factors such as stress, a common trigger in eczema is actually food.

2

ECZEMA-PRODUCING FOODS

The development of eczema is often related to the consumption of dairy products, wheat (bread, pasta, cookies, wheat-based breakfast cereals), red meat, citrus fruits, and eggs. Try eliminating these foods from your diet for three weeks. If your skin improves, you can be fairly confident that one of these food types is causing the problem. You could then try reintroducing these foods into your diet once every two days. A recurrence of symptoms is an indication that this is a likely trigger for your eczema.

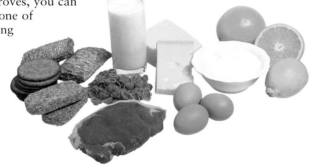

INFANTILE ECZEMA

Eczema that develops in infancy and early childhood is often due to a child's reaction to infant formulas based on cow's milk. In the first instance, it is worthwhile replacing these with soy-based formulas or cow's milk-based formulas that have been treated with enzymes to make them more digestible.

■ Consult your doctor about alternative formulas if you suspect your baby may have a problem with regular cow's milk formulas.

■ Older children with eczema should avoid all dairy products based on cow's milk including cheese and yogurt. Good substitutes include goat's and sheep's milk, soy milk, rice milk, and soybean cheese and yoghurt, all of which you should be able to find in a health food store.

■ It is worth noting that children often crave and become very attached to the foods to which they are most sensitive.

MILK SUBSTITUTES

Soy milk, rice milk, rye crackers, rice cakes, rice, rice pasta, and oat-based breakfast cereals are good alternatives to the main eczema-causing foods. There is a wide range of products to choose from in health food stores and, increasingly, in large supermarkets. For adults, cutting down on your consumption of dairy products also has other health benefits. By reducing your intake of unhealthful animal fats, you will be reducing your risk of heart disease.

TOPICAL TREATMENT

During an outbreak of eczema, apply a bland emollient cream to the rash to relieve itching and dryness.

2

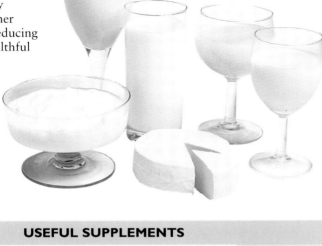

USEFUL SUPPLEMENTS

Supplement	Action	Dose
Gamma linoleic acid (GLA)	GLA, the active ingredient in evening primrose oil and starflower oil, is converted in the body into substances that have natural anti-inflammatory properties. GLA also helps to prevent dry skin, which is often a feature in eczema.	1–2 GLA capsules a day
Vitamin C	Vitamin C has an important role to play in skin health and healing. Women taking oral contraceptives should take a maximum daily dose of no more than 1000 mg.	1000 mg 2–3 times a day
Zinc	Like vitamin C, zinc helps with general skin healing and can help reduce eczema in a significant number of sufferers.	30–45 mg a day

PSORIASIS

Psoriasis is a chronic skin condition that normally gives rise to raised, red and scaly patches of skin, often on the knees, elbows, scalp, and behind the ears. The condition seems to be linked to rapid growth in the outer layers of the skin. Some psoriasis sufferers develop a form of arthritis known as psoriatic arthritis.

2

CAUSES

Although the precise cause of psoriasis is unknown, it does seem to be linked to certain factors. Psoriasis can tend to run in families, suggesting that a predisposition for the condition may be inherited. The development of psoriasis may also be linked to our emotional state, with a significant number of sufferers reporting that the condition started after a time of particular stress. Other theories regarding the cause of psoriasis include the consumption of too much animal fat in the diet, a malfunctioning immune system, and a buildup of toxins in the colon.

FOODS TO AVOID

Some foods seem to aggravate psoriasis, so you could try eliminating these foods for a month to see if this improves matters.

- Citrus fruits.

- Fried foods.

- Refined foods.

- Sugar.

- Meat and dairy products should be particularly avoided because they contain the substance arachidonic acid, which can make the psoriasis patches turn red and swell.

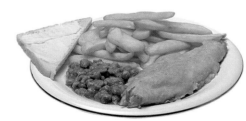

- Alcohol can put stress on the liver, reducing its ability to filter the blood efficiently. There is good evidence that alcohol consumption can considerably worsen psoriasis.

SUNLIGHT AND PSORIASIS

Exposure to ultraviolet light, either in the form of natural sunlight or from a sun bed, can significantly reduce the severity of psoriasis. Be sure not to overexpose your skin or let your skin burn.

FOODS TO EAT

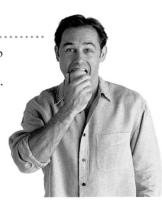

- You should eat plenty of high-fiber foods to help ensure regular bowel movements, reducing the likelihood that the colon will build up toxic waste.

- Fresh fruits.

- Vegetables.

- Oats.

- Water is also important to reduce toxicity. Drink at least 2½ pints of filtered or spring water each day.

2

USEFUL SUPPLEMENTS

Supplement	Action	Dose
Linseeds	An effective and convenient way to maintain bowel regularity and prevent toxicity is to add linseeds to your diet. Take either sprinkled on your cereal or with water.	1 tablespoon a day
Fish oil	Concentrated fish oil supplements have been shown to benefit psoriasis sufferers, although it can take several months of treatment before improvement is seen. 	1 g three times a day
Milk thistle	This herb is known to help support and strengthen the liver function, thereby reducing toxicity within the body. Milk thistle has other beneficial properties, including the ability to reduce inflammation and slow down excessive cell proliferation.	70–210 mg three times a day
Calendula	Creams based on this herb can be rubbed into dry and cracked lesions as often as required. This may help to reduce the pain and discomfort of psoriasis. 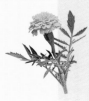	

COLD SORES

Cold sores are caused by the herpes virus and are characterized by single or multiple clusters of small blisters on a reddened base. Following initial infection, which may go unnoticed in childhood, the virus lies dormant in the body and is normally kept in check by the body's immune system. However, the virus can reactivate and cause cold sores from time to time, especially when we are run down and the immune system is weakened. Other trigger factors include minor infections (hence the term "cold sores"), exposure to heat, cold or strong sunlight, and excessive stress or tiredness. The appearance of a cold sore is usually preceded by a tingling sensation in the affected area.

FOODS TO AVOID

Certain foods tend to increase the chances of a recurrence of a cold sore because they contain an amino acid called arginine that stimulates replication of the herpes virus. Such foods include:

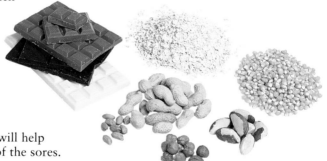

- Chocolate.

- Nuts (especially peanuts).

- Oats.

- Corn.

Avoiding these foods will help prevent a recurrence of the sores.

GENITAL HERPES

Cold sores and genital herpes are both caused by the herpes simplex virus (HSV). Genital herpes differs from cold sores in that the strain of the virus is different. Cold sores are usually caused by the herpes simplex virus 1 (HSV1), while genital herpes is usually caused by herpes simplex virus 2 (HSV2). The initial genital infection with HSV2 can cause painful enlargement of the glands (lymph nodes) in the groin in addition to one or more sores in the genital area itself. Like cold sores, genital herpes can tend to recur, particularly when the immune system is low. Because genital herpes is caused by a very similar virus to the one that causes cold sores, its treatment with natural remedies is the same. However, it is important to seek medical advice if you think you may have genital herpes.

FOODS THAT INCREASE IMMUNITY

Keep your diet based around foods that are rich in the immune-enhancing nutrients such as betacarotene, vitamin C, and zinc. Make sure you eat plenty of fresh fruits, vegetables, fish, and seeds. Avoid sugar as much as possible, since it is known to dampen immune activity.

2

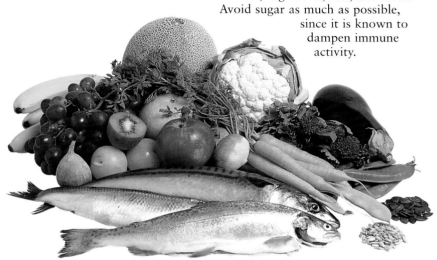

USEFUL SUPPLEMENTS

Supplement	Action	Dose
Lysine	Taking the amino acid lysine when you feel the first signs of a cold sore can often stop an attack from developing, since it interferes with the growth of the herpes virus.	1 g three times a day
Vitamin C	Vitamin C can be taken in conjunction with lysine at the first signs of an attack to help prevent a cold sore from developing. Women taking oral contraceptives should take no more than 1000 mg a day.	1 g three times a day
Echinacea	Echinacea can help to improve immune function and increase resistance to the herpes virus.	Follow the instructions on the label
Lemon balm	This herb has antiviral properties. Application of a cream containing lemon balm extract to the blisters can speed healing and help to prevent further outbreaks.	Follow the instructions on the label

CATARACTS

L ight is focused onto the seeing part of the eye (the retina) by the lens, which is composed of a transparent, jellylike material. Sometimes, the lens of the eye can lose its transparent quality, leading to a gradual deterioration in vision. This condition is known as a cataract, and it may affect one or both eyes. The conventional medical approach to an advanced cataract is to remove the lens surgically and replace it with a synthetic one.

2

PREVENTING LENS DAMAGE

Cataract formation seems to be related to damage to proteins in the lens of the eye by destructive molecules in the body called free radicals. One of the factors that encourages free radical production is sunlight, so you can make an important contribution to the prevention of the condition by protecting your eyes when you are in strong sunlight by wearing sunglasses that effectively block ultraviolet light.

COUNTERING FREE RADICAL ACTIVITY

Free radical damage in the body is increased by many lifestyle factors including stress, smoking, and overconsumption of fat and alcohol. To reduce your risk of developing a cataract or to help prevent a worsening of one already present, it is wise to avoid these factors as much as possible.
     Free radical damage in the body is counteracted by antioxidant nutrients such as betacarotene, vitamins A, C, and E, and the mineral selenium. Make sure you eat an abundance of foods rich in these nutrients including fresh fruits, vegetables, and whole grains such as whole-wheat bread and pasta, and brown rice.

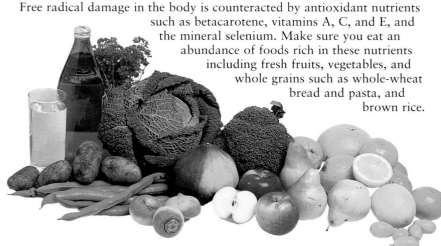

USEFUL SUPPLEMENTS

Cataract sufferers often benefit from taking antioxidant nutrients in supplement form. Some eye specialists in the U.S. claim that treating people with antioxidant nutrients can halt cataract development and even improve vision in a significant number of patients.

Supplement	Action	Dose
Betacarotene	Antioxidant action counters the damaging effects of free radicals.	25,000–50,000 IU a day
Vitamin C	Antioxidant action counters the damaging effects of free radicals. Women taking oral contraceptives should take no more than 1000 mg a day.	1000 mg twice a day
Vitamin E	Antioxidant. One study noted that people with low levels of vitamin E in their blood are nearly twice as likely to develop cataracts as people with normal levels.	400 IU a day
Selenium	Antioxidant action counters the damaging effects of free radicals.	200 mcg a day
Zinc	This mineral is important for healthy vision.	30–45 mg a day
Bilberry	In addition to the standard antioxidant nutrients, taking the more specialized nutrient bilberry may help prevent or slow down cataract formation. Bilberry has been used by herbalists for years to treat a variety of eye conditions including cataracts. In one study, bilberry extract in combination with vitamin E stopped cataract development in a very high percentage of elderly sufferers.	40–80 mg three times a day

2

MACULAR DEGENERATION

L ight from the outside world is focused onto a structure at the back of the eye called the retina. In macular degeneration, there is destruction of the macula, a particular part of the retina that is crucial for vision. This small spot on the retina is responsible for fine vision and for distinguishing color. Damage to the macula can severely impair the ability to see. Blurred vision, visual distortion, and dark spots in the field of vision are typical symptoms. Approximately a quarter of people over the age of 65 have at least the first stages of macular degeneration, and it is the leading cause of irreversible loss of vision in people over the age of 60.

DIETARY RISK FACTORS

Macular degeneration may be triggered by the effects of damaging, destructive molecules called free radicals on the blood vessels. People who eat few fresh fruits and vegetables and who have high levels of cholesterol in their bloodstream seem to be at increased risk. This may be because high cholesterol levels can cause clogging of the vessels that supply blood to the eyes, thereby increasing the risk of damage. To reduce your risk of developing this condition, it is important to minimize your intake of red meat and dairy products, including butter, cream, cheese, and eggs. Avoid fried foods and convenience foods, which are often high in fat.

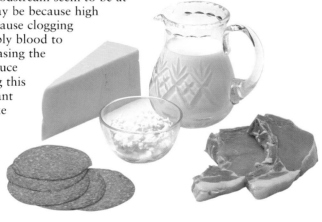

LIFESTYLE FACTORS

Free radical damage in the body is increased by lifestyle factors including stress, smoking, and the overconsumption of alcohol. To reduce your risk of developing macular degeneration, it is wise to avoid these factors as much as possible.

FOODS TO EAT

Free radicals are neutralized by substances called antioxidants such as the nutrient betacarotene. One study showed that eating betacarotene-rich foods such as red and orange peppers, apricots, cantaloupe, kale, and spinach helped reduce risk of macular degeneration. Make sure you include plenty of antioxidant rich foods in your diet. Zinc is another nutrient that has been shown to be important for the health of the retina. Dietary sources of this mineral include fish, seafood, and whole grains such as whole-wheat bread.

2

USEFUL SUPPLEMENTS

Supplement	Action	Dose
Lutein and zeaxanthin	These two nutrients are related to betacarotene and appear to have important roles in protecting the macula from free radical damage. They can often be obtained in a combined preparation for eye health.	Follow the instructions on the label
Vitamin C	Studies have shown that people who take vitamin C in supplement form are less likely to develop macular degeneration than those who don't. This protective effect is probably achieved through vitamin C's antioxidant properties. Women taking oral contraceptives should take a maximum daily dose of no more than 1000 mg.	1000 mg twice a day
Zinc	Zinc is essential to the metabolic function of some cells in the retina, and regular supplements have been shown to slow loss of vision resulting from macular degeneration.	45–60 mg a day

GLAUCOMA

Each eye is filled with a fluid that is essential for maintaining its normal shape. Sometimes the pressure in one or both eyes can increase, and this gives rise to a condition known as glaucoma. Ninety percent of glaucoma cases are of the type known as "chronic glaucoma." In this condition, there are usually no symptoms until significant elevations in eye pressure are present. When the pressure of fluids in the eye reaches high levels, a gradual loss of peripheral vision – sometimes called "tunnel vision" – is experienced. Chronic glaucoma can lead to damage to the major nerve in the eye, causing gradual loss of vision over time.

THE ROLE OF CAFFEINE

There is some evidence that caffeine can raise the pressure in the eyes. Cut out any caffeinated beverages and chocolate from your diet. Opt for naturally caffeine-free herb tea and decaffeinated coffee and tea instead.

Warning

The acute form of glaucoma requires immediate medical attention to prevent permanent loss of vision. Call your doctor at once if you have severe eye pain and blurred vision.

USEFUL SUPPLEMENTS

Supplement	Action	Dose
Vitamin C	Vitamin C has been shown to reduce pressure in the eye in those suffering from chronic glaucoma. Women taking oral contraceptives should take a maximum daily dose of no more than 1000 mg.	1000 mg three times a day
Bioflavonoids	Bioflavonoid compounds are found in fruits and vegetables (especially the pith of citrus fruits) and are believed to help reduce eye pressure.	500 mg twice a day

Muscles, Bones, and Teeth

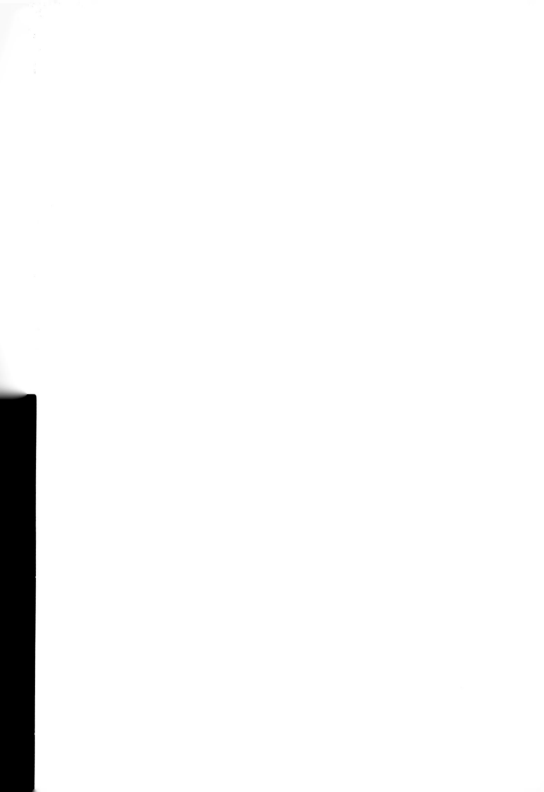

MUSCLES, BONES AND TEETH

Movement is a natural part of human existence. Whether we want to comb our hair or run a marathon, we depend on the health of our bones, joints and muscles. If any of these crucial areas becomes diseased, our ability to live life to the full can be curtailed. This chapter looks at some of the major bones and joint conditions such as arthritis, gout and osteoporosis. Natural medicine has much to offer in the treatment of these conditions. Dietary changes and nutritional supplements offer relief for conditions that affect our mobility, without the side effects associated with the use of painkilling medications. In addition, this chapter looks at the dietary factors and nutrients that are important for dental health.

3

SPORTS PERFORMANCE

Food is the fuel that drives our body's machinery. Eating a healthy diet based on low-fat, nutritious foods such as fresh fruit, vegetables and wholegrains can go a long way to ensuring the body gets the fuel it needs for optimum performance. However, taking additional nutrients may improve performance and recovery.

MAINTAINING ENERGY

Blood sugar levels are topped up during exercise from glycogen stores in the liver and muscles. If glycogen is not replaced between training sessions, glycogen levels in the body can get depleted over a period of time. The way to maintain glycogen levels is to eat a diet rich in healthy carbohydrates from fresh fruit, potatoes, brown rice, wholewheat pasta, oats and wholemeal bread.

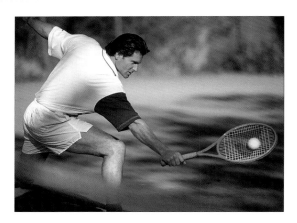

USEFUL SUPPLEMENTS

Supplement	Action	Dose
Anti-oxidant formulation	Damaging molecules called free radicals are constantly being produced as a by-product of metabolism. These have been implicated in the soreness and fatigue we may feel for some time after exercise. Anti-oxidant nutrients such as the vitamins A, C and E and the mineral selenium neutralize free radicals and may therefore reduce the negative effects of exercise on the body.	Follow the instructions on the label
B-complex	The B-complex vitamins play an essential role in the reactions that unlock energy from food. Additional quantities of B vitamins (particularly vitamins B_2, B_5 and B_6) can boost energy levels.	50 mg of vitamins B_1–B_6 a day.

Supplement	Action	Dose
Coenzyme Q10	The processes that generate energy from food take place in minute power-houses in each cell called the mitochondria. Here, energy in food is converted into molecules of a substance called ATP which the body then uses to generate energy. Coenzyme Q10 (also known as Co-Q10 and ubiquinone) is a key catalyst in the process that generates ATP. Supplementing with Coenzyme Q10 is well known to improve energy levels and increase our capacity for physical work.	30–50 mg three times a day
Siberian ginseng	Siberian ginseng has been used in Chinese medicine for over 2000 years, both as an energy booster and an immune system enhancer. The active ingredients in Siberian ginseng support the function of the body's chief organs responsible for dealing with stress – the adrenal glands. Siberian ginseng's effects are quite similar to those of caffeine, and studies have shown it can sharpen the mind as well as improve physical energy. It is generally recommended that Siberian ginseng be used on a cyclical basis with treatment periods of six to eight weeks interspersed with breaks lasting two weeks.	300–400 mg of solid concentrated standardized extract a day or 2–3 g of dried powder a day

Caution

Siberian ginseng may cause mild, transient diarrhoea and insomnia if taken too close to bedtime. It should not be used by those suffering from high blood pressure. It is also not recommended if you are pregnant or breastfeeding.

Supplement	Action	Dose
Branched-chain amino acids	Branched-chain amino acids (BCAAs) can be useful for athletes who do not consume enough protein in their diets. BCAA supplements may reduce muscle loss and speed muscle gain.	Follow the instructions on the label
Creatine monohydrate	Creatine assists in the production of energy and muscle-building processes. In tests, it has been found to increase athletic performance.	Follow the instructions on the label

3

CRAMP

Cramp is a painful spasm in a muscle caused by excessive or prolonged contraction of muscle fibres, often in the calves, feet or back of the thighs. Cramps usually last for a few moments, but can quite commonly occur at night and disrupt sleep. Another common time for cramp is during or just after exercise. Here, cramp is thought to be related to a build-up of lactic acid and other waste products of metabolism in the muscles.

IS LACK OF SALT A CAUSE OF CRAMP?

It is often thought that cramp is due to a deficiency of salt (sodium chloride) in the diet. However, this is actually a very rare cause of cramp and, in fact, most of us eat far too much salt. Cramp is more commonly related to a deficiency of calcium, magnesium or potassium, minerals that are involved in the conduction of nerve signals in the muscles.

3

PREVENTING CRAMP THROUGH DIET

It is important to increase your consumption of foods that are rich in calcium, magnesium and potassium. Eating more of these foods can sometimes be all it takes to stop recurrent cramp attacks.

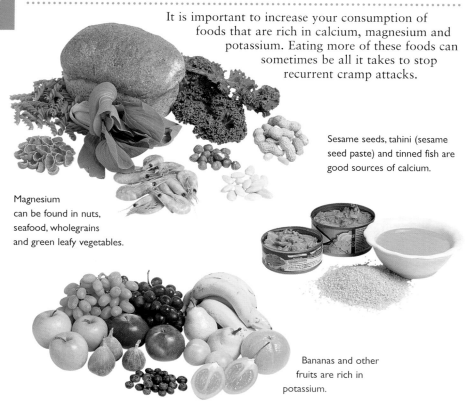

Sesame seeds, tahini (sesame seed paste) and tinned fish are good sources of calcium.

Magnesium can be found in nuts, seafood, wholegrains and green leafy vegetables.

Bananas and other fruits are rich in potassium.

STRETCHING

The regular stretching of muscles may help prevent cramp. Many individuals find that the stretching of the calf muscles prior to getting into bed can cut down the frequency of night cramp attacks.

RESTLESS LEGS

Restless legs is a syndrome characterized by uncomfortable tickling, burning, prickling or aching sensations in the muscles of the legs. Sufferers usually find that symptoms develop at night while they are in bed. This condition is thought to affect as many as 15 per cent of the population. You should avoid coffee and tea because caffeine can often trigger symptoms. Restless legs is also associated with smoking – so if you smoke you should consider stopping or at least cutting down.

Supplement	Dose
Magnesium	500 mg a day
Vitamin E	300 IU a day

3

USEFUL SUPPLEMENTS

Supplement	Action	Dose
Calcium	Calcium in important for the conduction of nerve signals in the muscles. Deficiency of this mineral may contribute to cramp.	1000–1500 mg with evening meal
Magnesium	Magnesium, like calcium (above), is needed for the normal transmission of nerve signals in the muscles.	500–750 mg with evening meal
Vitamin E	Vitamin E may be a useful adjunct to calcium and magnesium supplementation because it can increase blood flow to the muscles. This seems to have a normalizing effect on muscle function and can help prevent cramp.	300 IU with evening meal

CARPAL TUNNEL SYNDROME

Carpal tunnel syndrome (CTS) is a condition where one of the major nerves that supplies the hand – the median nerve – becomes trapped under a band of fibrous tissue (the flexor retinaculum) as it runs through the wrist. The median nerve carries sensation from the thumb, index, middle and thumb side of the ring finger. It also controls muscular function in some of the hand's muscles. Typical symptoms of CTS include numbness, tingling and weakness in the affected hand(s).

CAUSES OF CARPAL TUNNEL SYNDROME

Carpal tunnel syndrome occurs most frequently in the following groups:

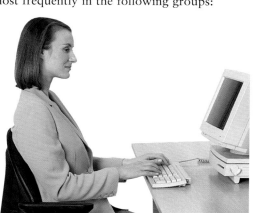

- People who spend a large proportion of their time working at a computer keyboard.

- Those prone to fluid retention, in particular pregnant women, women using the oral contraceptive pill, and those suffering from premenstrual syndrome.

- Those suffering from rheumatoid arthritis or an underactive thyroid gland.

TESTING FOR CARPAL TUNNEL SYNDROME

A diagnosis of CTS can be confirmed by measuring the passage of nerve impulses through the median nerve to the muscles of the hand. However, there is a simple test which you can do yourself which can help ascertain whether the symptoms that you have are due to CTS.

- Hold your hands out with your palms up. Bend each of your fingers at the two outer joints only, leaving the joints where your fingers meet your palm straight. Bring the tips of your fingers down to the palms of your hands, right to the crease that separates the fingers from the hands. If any of these 16 joints cannot be bent completely without pain, then CTS is suspected.

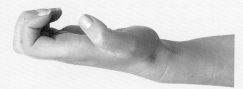

3

SURGICAL TREATMENT

The conventional medical approach to carpal tunnel syndrome includes splinting, rest, painkillers and surgery. Surgery has mixed results and, in a proportion of patients, scar tissue forms around the operation site causing compression of the median nerve and a recurrence of the original symptoms.

REDUCING SALT INTAKE

On a dietary level the most important thing you can do is to avoid salt because it can promote water retention which increases swelling of the tissues around the nerves in the wrist. Do not add any salt to food during cooking or at the table. It may help to cut down slowly so that your taste adapts to lower salt levels gradually.

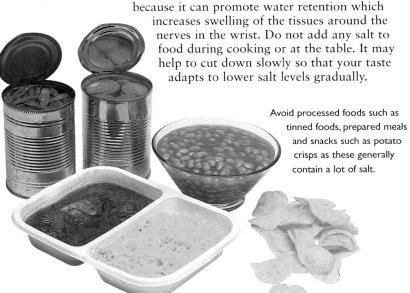

Avoid processed foods such as tinned foods, prepared meals and snacks such as potato crisps as these generally contain a lot of salt.

3

USEFUL SUPPLEMENTS

Supplement	Action	Dose
Vitamin B$_6$	The nutrient that seems to be most effective in treating carpal tunnel syndrome is vitamin B$_6$. Several studies demonstrate significant relief for a large proportion of sufferers with B$_6$ supplementation. Taking 100 mg a day for three months may well relieve symptoms.	100 mg a day

OSTEOARTHRITIS

Osteoarthritis is the most common problem affecting the joints and typically causes pain, swelling and stiffness, particularly in the hip or knee. The condition is associated with a slow, progressive wearing down of the cartilage that cushions the joints, and a loss of fluid that is responsible for keeping the joints lubricated. The older we get, the more likely we are to develop osteoarthritis, with six out of ten of individuals over the age of 60 being affected.

PAINKILLERS

The conventional medical approach to osteoarthritis revolves around the use of painkillers and surgery. Non-steroidal anti-inflammatory drugs such as ibuprofen are often prescribed for osteoarthritis. While these may be effective in treating the pain of arthritis, there is some evidence that their use is related to an increased rate of the degeneration of joint cartilage. Another downside to non-steroidal anti-inflammatory drugs is their side-effects: inflammation and ulcers in the lining of the digestive tract and nausea are common and sometimes serious complications. Natural methods of treating osteoarthritis through diet and nutritional supplements can often reduce the need for painkillers and therefore the risk of side effects.

FOODS THAT AGGRAVATE ARTHRITIS

The pain and inflammation of osteoarthritis seem to be made worse by eating certain foods. Common problem foods include:

- Dairy products.

- Red meat.

- Citrus fruits.

- Foods that belong to the nightshade family (potatoes, aubergines, red and green peppers and tomatoes).

Reduce your intake of all these foods.

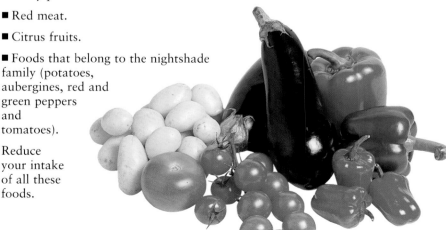

3

FOODS THAT HELP

Eating plenty of fresh fruit and vegetables will help restore alkalinity to the body which can help reduce symptoms in all forms of arthritis. Drink several cups of ginger tea each day as ginger has natural pain-relieving and anti-inflammatory properties. You can make this simply and cheaply at home by steeping freshly chopped ginger in hot water. Add a little honey to taste.

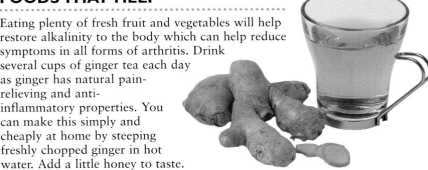

CONTROL YOUR WEIGHT

Carrying excess weight increases the strain on damaged joints. If you are overweight, try to lose the excess. Take regular, gentle exercise such as swimming and walking, and reduce your intake of sugary and fatty foods.

3

USEFUL SUPPLEMENTS

Supplement	Action	Dose
Glucosamine sulphate	All tissues, including cartilage, are constantly regenerated by the body. It is thought that in osteoarthritis, however, the cartilage degenerates more quickly than it regenerates. One of the main building blocks of cartilage is glucosamine, and there is evidence that taking it in supplement form can stimulate healing and repair of joint cartilage. Glucosamine has been proven to be as effective as non-steroidal anti-inflammatory drugs in the treatment of osteoarthritis and works by stimulating healing rather than by merely suppressing pain.	500 mg three times a day
Fish oil	Fish oil supplements that are rich in the omega-3 essential fats known as EPA and DHA are often very effective in relieving the symptoms of osteoarthritis. EPA and DHA reduce inflammation in the joints, and increase the production of joint lubricating fluid.	1 g three times a day

RHEUMATOID ARTHRITIS

R heumatoid arthritis is an inflammatory condition characterized by inflammation in the joints of the fingers, toes, wrists or other joints of the body. The affected joints become swollen and stiff and may become deformed in the long term. The disease usually comes in waves, with painful periods being interspersed with times when sufferers are relatively symptom-free. The disease usually starts in early adulthood or middle age but can sometimes start in childhood. Rheumatoid arthritis affects 2–3 per cent of the population and about 75 per cent of sufferers are women.

WHAT CAUSES RHEUMATOID ARTHRITIS

Rheumatoid arthritis is what is known as an "auto-immune" disease. The body's immune system mounts an attack against the body's own tissues causing inflammation and long-term damage. In the case of rheumatoid arthritis, the part of the body that is affected is the tissue that lines the joints known as the "synovium".

3

THE FOOD TRIGGERS

While the cause of rheumatoid arthritis is not known for sure, there is some evidence that it can be triggered by food. It is thought that partially digested food leaks through the intestinal wall into the bloodstream, going on to trigger immune reactions in the joints. Common culprits in these reactions include wheat, corn, dairy products and citrus fruits. A significant number of rheumatoid arthritis sufferers find that identifying and eliminating problem foods from the diet can lead to significant improvement in their symptoms.

FOODS TO AVOID

There are some foods that we may eat on a day-to-day basis that seem to promote the processes that cause inflammation in the body. Common examples are:
■ Red meat.

■ Sugar.

■ Coffee.

■ Tea.

Cutting back on these foods or eliminating them altogether may therefore help to reduce the symptoms of rheumatoid arthritis.

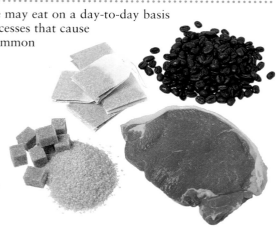

ANTI-INFLAMMATORY FOODS

Eating plenty of foods that tend to have an anti-inflammatory effect in the body may help to reduce pain and inflammation in the joints. Healthy fats, also known as essential fatty acids, in the diet are metabolized in the body into substances that have natural anti-inflammatory properties. Foods that are rich in these healthy fats include oily fish such as mackerel, salmon and trout, olive oil and pumpkin, sunflower and sesame seeds. Increase the amount of these foods in your diet.

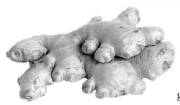

Another food that helps reduce inflammation naturally is ginger. This can be added to stir-fries and other dishes. A convenient way to get the benefit of ginger is to take it as a tea. This is made by steeping some freshly sliced or grated root ginger in hot water.

3

USEFUL SUPPLEMENTS		
Supplement	**Action**	**Dose**
Fish oil	Fish oils that are high in the essential fats EPA and DHA have a natural anti-inflammatory effect in the body and can therefore help reduce the joint pain and swelling characteristic of rheumatoid arthritis.	I g three times a day
Ginger capsules	Renowned for its anti-inflammatory properties, ginger has been shown to provide relief for a significant number of sufferers of rheumatoid arthritis.	200–400 mg three times a day
Bromelain	This extract of pineapple has potent anti-inflammatory activity when taken on an empty stomach.	150–450 mg three times a day on an empty stomach

GOUT

Gout is a type of arthritis that is caused by the accumulation of uric acid in the body. Crystals of uric acid can form in a joint – usually the big toe – and this can lead to intense pain and inflammation. Gout tends to occur in middle or old age, and nine out of ten sufferers are men. Gout is traditionally thought to be the consequence of consuming too much rich food and alcohol. However, not all cases of gout are due to dietary over-indulgence, with many cases occurring in individuals who do not eat an excess of rich foods. In these cases there may be a problem with the excretion of uric acid from the body.

URIC ACID PRODUCING FOODS

Uric acid is actually a breakdown product of a class of substances known as purines. It is important for sufferers to avoid all foods that contain a high concentration of purines including:

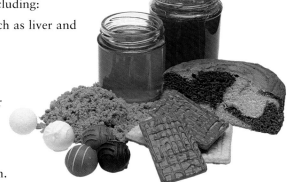

- Meat and organ meats such as liver and kidney.

- Seafood.

- Beans, peas and lentils.

Reduce your intake of sugar as this can increase the level of uric acid in the blood. Also avoid honey, jams, biscuits, cakes and confectionery for this reason.

3

OTHER FORMS OF GOUT

While, classically, gout is thought to be a condition which affects the big toe, the fact is that crystals of uric acid can deposit anywhere in the body giving rise to symptoms. It is not uncommon for widespread deposition of uric acid in the joints and tendons to give rise to a condition known as "gouty arthritis". Commonly affected joints include the knee, ankle, wrist, foot and small joints of the hand. Natural treatments for gouty arthritis are the same as those for gout affecting a single joint.

Uric acid crystals can also accumulate in the kidneys. This can lead to kidney stones and, in severe cases, long-term damage to the kidneys. While natural treatments can help, close medical supervision is required if the kidneys are affected.

BENEFICIAL FOODS

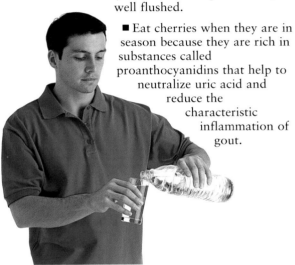

- Eat plenty of fresh fruits and vegetables which will help to alkalinize your system and help neutralize the effect of the uric acid in the body.

- Drink 1–1½ litres of filtered or still mineral water each day to help dilute uric acid in the system and to keep the kidneys well flushed.

- Eat cherries when they are in season because they are rich in substances called proanthocyanidins that help to neutralize uric acid and reduce the characteristic inflammation of gout.

ALCOHOL AND GOUT

Excessive consumption of alcohol, particularly port, is popularly linked with susceptibility to gout. In fact, gout can occur in those who never drink alcohol. However, it is true that alcohol can aggravate the condition and it should therefore be avoided.

3

USEFUL SUPPLEMENTS

Supplement	Action	Dose
Cherry extract	Pill or powdered extracts are an all-year-round alternative to fresh cherries.	Follow the instructions on the label
Celery seed	This herbal supplement may help reduce the symptoms of gout because it has natural anti-inflammatory and neutralizing properties.	Follow the instructions on the label
Bromelain	This extract of pineapple has potent anti-inflammatory activity when taken on an empty stomach.	150–450 mg 3 times a day on an empty stomach

OSTEOPOROSIS

Bone is living tissue and is constantly being renewed and replaced in the body. Thinning bones, or osteoporosis, come about when bone tissue is broken down faster than it is formed. When this happens the bones can become weakened and this increases the chances of fracture, especially in the spine and hips.

WHAT CAUSES OSTEOPOROSIS

Osteoporosis is much more common in women than men and is usually related to falling oestrogen levels after the menopause. Sex hormones play an important role in bone formation. There is also a hereditary link, with increased risk being found in individuals who have an affected close blood relative. Immobility, for example, as a result of long-term illness, can also lead to bone loss. Although osteoporosis is to some degree a natural part of the ageing process, there is much that may be done to help slow its progress.

REDUCING BONE LOSS

Studies have shown that gentle weight-bearing exercise reduces bone loss and may even increase bone density. Good forms of exercise include brisk walking, light jogging and light weight-lifting. Aim to get about 30 minutes of exercise each day. On a dietary level it is important for you to avoid sugar, red meat and fizzy drinks as these tend to speed up the rate at which calcium is lost from the bone. At the same time, increase your intake of foods that are rich in calcium and magnesium, both of which are essential for healthy bone formation. Green leafy vegetables, sardines, mackerel, seafood and sesame seeds are all good sources of these essential minerals.

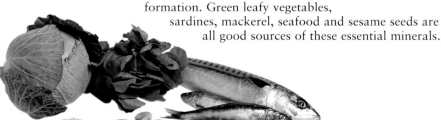

USEFUL SUPPLEMENTS

Supplement	Action	Dose
Calcium	Since the principle nutrient in bone is calcium, there has been a lot of research looking at the link between calcium consumption and osteoporosis and there is good evidence that women with a high intake of calcium are at reduced risk of osteoporosis.	Men and pre-menopaual women: 500 mg a day Post-menopausal women 1000 mg a day
Magnesium	The more magnesium there is in the diet, the higher bone density tends to be. Magnesium has an important part to play in the building of bone in the body. It activates an enzyme which is involved in laying down calcium in bone. People with osteoporosis may have a reduced level of magnesium in their bones and often show evidence of magnesium deficiency.	500 mg a day
Vitamin D	Along with calcium and magnesium, vitamin D is one of the key nutrients involved in bone formation. Lack of exposure to sunlight and/or a poor diet can create a need for supplements.	400 IU a day
Boron	Boron is a trace mineral which has a very important part to play in the health and strength of the bones. Its presence in the body seems to slow down the rate at which calcium and magnesium are excreted. In addition, boron can increase the level of oestrogen in the blood, which then may have a positive impact on bone formation.	1–3 mg a day
Vitamin C	Adequate amounts of vitamin C are required in the body to activate the enzyme necessary for the manufacture of collagen, a major component of bone.	500 mg a day

3

DENTAL HEALTH

Dental decay (caries) is one of the most prevalent health problems in the Western world. There is no doubt that dental problems are linked to nutritional factors and these come into play even before we are born. Even though a baby's first teeth do not appear until about six months of age, teeth start to develop as early as the seventh week of pregnancy. and calcification of teeth begins in about the fourth month of pregnancy. The mother's diet during pregnancy therefore has an important influence on the future development of her child's teeth. Women should ensure an adequate intake of calcium during pregnancy for this reason. (See also Pregnancy support, page 108.)

3

GROWING TEETH

After birth, the best food for strong and healthy teeth is breast milk. What is more, a breastfed baby is much less likely to suffer from tooth decay caused by a pooling of milk in the mouth. This is a common occurrence in babies who fall asleep taking milk from a bottle. Studies also show that breastfed infants are less likely to need orthodontic treatment later in life. After weaning, you should avoid giving your baby foods and drinks containing sugar, which can damage tooth enamel. Even natural sugars in fruit juice can cause problems, so make sure you dilute adequately any juices you offer your baby.

Warning

During pregnancy it is important for women to avoid taking antibiotics based on tetracycline. These can cause permanent discoloration of a baby's teeth. Tetracycline can also cause discoloration of the permanent teeth if given to children during the time these teeth are forming (3–12 years of age).

FLUORIDE

It is well known that this mineral can reduce the rate of dental decay in children. Fluoride is incorporated into the tooth enamel, making it more resistant to decay. It appears to be most beneficial for young children whose teeth are just developing. In many areas fluoride is routinely added to the water supply and it is an ingredient in the vast majority of toothpastes.

DENTAL CARE

Regular brushing is one of the most important contributions you can make to dental health. Regular removal of food residues helps to prevent the developement of tooth decay (caries) and gum disease. Teach your children to brush their teeth properly and supervise tooth-brushing until you are sure they can do it thoroughly for themselves.

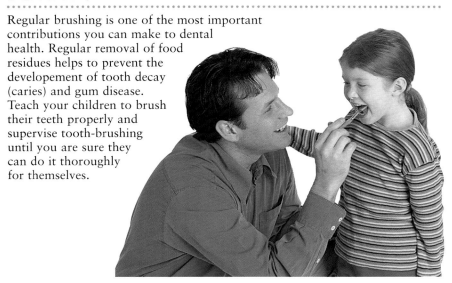

3

EATING FOR DENTAL HEALTH THROUGHOUT LIFE

Throughout childhood, adolescence and adulthood it remains important to avoid sugar in the diet. Sticky or chewy forms of sugar such as toffee and caramel are worse for your teeth than less adherent forms of sugar. But all sweet foods encourage the formation of acids that cause decay. Include in your daily diet plenty of non-acidic, hard and fibrous foods that help to cleanse the teeth. These include cucumber, celery and lettuce.

    How we eat is also important for dental health. Frequent sipping of sweet drinks and snacking on sugary foods ensures that levels of damaging acids in the mouth remain constantly high, increasing the risk of decay. If you are hungry between meals, choose a low-sugar snack instead. Quench your thirst with plain water or other unsweetened drinks.

USEFUL SUPPLEMENTS		
Supplement	**Action**	**Dose**
Clove oil	Clove oil has a long history of use as a painkiller for toothache. Apply it directly to the tooth until you can see your dentist.	As often as needed
Calcium	This mineral is essential for tooth formation in children. Supplements may be helpful if the diet is low in natural sources.	200–500 mg a day

GUM DISEASE

Inflammation and sometimes infection in the gum line is known as gingivitis. Gingivitis is responsible for about 10 per cent of all dental extractions. Another common gum problem is bleeding gums, a prime cause of which is over-zealous or too frequent brushing. Gentle brushing twice a day with a soft toothbrush may help to reduce damage to the gums and prevent bleeding.

DIETARY MEASURES

It is important for the health of your gums to minimize consumption of fizzy drinks, sweets, sugar and refined carbohydrates like white bread, all of which tend to worsen any gum problem. Eat a diet rich in fresh fruits and vegetables and wholegrain starches such as wholemeal bread and brown rice.

STRENGTHENING THE BLOOD VESSELS

3

Sometimes a tendency for gums to bleed can be caused by a weakness in the tiny blood vessels of the gums themselves. This can indicate vitamin C deficiency. Taking extra vitamin C and certain nutrients known as bioflavonoids which are found in fresh fruits and vegetables can strengthen these blood vessels and prevent bleeding.

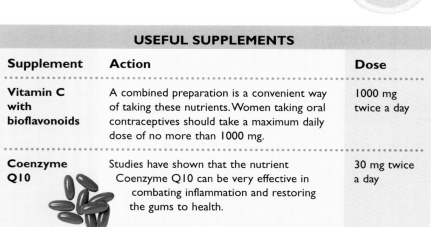

USEFUL SUPPLEMENTS		
Supplement	**Action**	**Dose**
Vitamin C with bioflavonoids	A combined preparation is a convenient way of taking these nutrients. Women taking oral contraceptives should take a maximum daily dose of no more than 1000 mg.	1000 mg twice a day
Coenzyme Q10	Studies have shown that the nutrient Coenzyme Q10 can be very effective in combating inflammation and restoring the gums to health.	30 mg twice a day

The Immune System

4

THE IMMUNE SYSTEM

The immune system is constantly protecting us from attack by microorganisms such as bacteria and viruses. If our immune system is weakened, our resistance to infection is lowered, and harmful organisms are more likely to take a hold in the body. The immune system also scavenges the body for cancer cells, and there is some evidence that poor immunity may increase our risk of certain cancers. By maintaining an adequate intake of the right nutrients and supplements, you can strengthen your immune system and increase its ability to fight disease.

Sometimes the immune cells are over-reactive, giving rise to allergic conditions such as hay fever and asthma. Here again, dietary changes and well-chosen supplements may offer effective and safe solutions to these problems.

COLDS AND FLU

Colds and flu are caused by viruses that are spread when we are in close proximity to others. Most of the time, undesirable germs are kept at bay by our immune system, which is constantly on the lookout for anything that may pose a threat to the body. However, if the immune system is weak, resistance is reduced and we are more likely to go down with a cold or flu.

FEEDING THE IMMUNE SYSTEM

Sugar tends to depress immune function and so is best avoided. Instead, your diet should be based on foods rich in nutrients such as betacarotene, vitamins A and C, and the mineral zinc, all of which are known to improve immune function. Increasing your intake of fresh fruits, vegetables, seeds, and fish will help ensure a good intake of these nutrients. Avoid juice "drinks," since they usually have excessive amounts of sugar added.

EXERCISE AND MENTAL ATTITUDE

Regular, moderate exercise can help the immune system function more efficiently – you should aim to take about 30 minutes of exercise most days. However, while moderate exercise can improve immune function, strenuous and prolonged exercise may have the reverse effect, so it is important not to overdo it.

Another important influence on immune function is our mental attitude. Studies have shown that negative emotions such as anger can depress immune function while more positive emotions actually strengthen it. Keeping a positive mental attitude is therefore important in warding off infection.

4

AT THE FIRST SIGN OF A COLD

If you take active steps at the first sign of a cold – for example, when you notice a sore or dry throat or you start to sneeze – you may be able to prevent it from developing or at least minimize its severity.

■ Drink plenty of clear fluids such as plain water and herb teas.

■ Take the supplements listed below.

■ Eat light but nutritious foods. Avoid dairy products, which may encourage mucus production.

■ Rest and keep warm.

USEFUL SUPPLEMENTS

Supplement	Action	Dose
Vitamin C	Vitamin C has potent immune-stimulating and antiviral properties. The main potential side effect of large doses of vitamin C is a loosening of the bowels. If this occurs, the dose of vitamin C should be reduced. Women taking oral contraceptives should take no more than 1000 mg a day.	1 g twice a day (prevention) 1 g every 2 hours (to speed recovery)
Zinc	Zinc has powerful immune-stimulating properties. Taking it in supplement form may well help to prevent infections in the long term. In addition, zinc lozenges have been found to be very effective in improving symptoms and speeding recovery from viral illnesses.	30–45 mg a day
Echinacea	Echinacea is the extract of the purple coneflower. This herb can help improve immune efficiency and may help to speed recovery from colds or flu. Seek medical advice if you have tuberculosis, multiple sclerosis, or systemic lupus erythematosus.	Follow the instructions on the label
Garlic	Garlic, famed for its beneficial effects on the heart and circulation, also has natural antibiotic properties. Studies show that garlic increases the number of immune cells in the body.	500 mg of garlic extract twice a day

4

HAY FEVER

Hay fever is caused by an allergic reaction to pollen causing the release of histamine around the nose and eyes. Characteristic symptoms include red, itchy eyes, and a runny or congested nose. The timing of the onset of hay fever symptoms gives a clue to which type of pollen is the problem. Symptoms coming on in spring point to tree pollen as the culprit, while early to mid summer is the peak time for grass pollen.

MEDICAL TREATMENTS

The conventional medical approach to hay fever generally consists of three types of medication: antihistamines that block the release of the histamine responsible for swelling and congestion; steroid-based nasal sprays; and decongestants such as ephedrine. Many people dislike taking such treatments for extended periods because of their unpleasant side effects and often gain benefit from dietary changes and natural supplements that significantly reduce or even eliminate the need for such medication.

REDUCING THE SYMPTOMS

Although hay fever is essentially caused by a reaction to pollen, certain foods are known to worsen the symptoms by triggering the immune system. Try avoiding the following foods:

- Wheat.
- Dairy products such as cow's milk and cheese.
- Strawberries.

Soy and rice milk and goat's cheese are good alternatives to cow's milk and cheese, while oats, rice, rice crackers, rye bread, and rye crackers are good substitutes for wheat.

4

PERENNIAL RHINITIS

While hay fever is essentially a seasonal complaint, allergic symptoms in some individuals can occur all year round. This is a condition known as "perennial rhinitis." The trigger factors in perennial rhinitis are very varied, but include dog and cat hair, feathers, the house dust mite, and environmental chemicals. Despite the different triggers, hay fever and perennial rhinitis have the same underlying processes and can therefore be treated in the same dietary way.

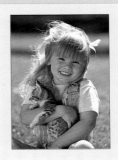

USEFUL SUPPLEMENTS

Supplement	Action	Dose
Vitamin C	Vitamin C has a natural antihistamine effect in the body and can therefore help to reduce and sometimes even eliminate the symptoms of hay fever. Women taking oral contraceptives should take no more than 1000 mg a day.	1000 mg three times a day
Quercetin	Quercetin is a substance from a group of nutrients known as bioflavonoids. There is some evidence that quercetin can reduce the release of histamine from immune system cells known as mast cells. In this way, quercetin can significantly reduce the symptoms of hay fever.	400 mg 3–4 times a day
Bromelain	Quercetin's effects seem to be most potent when coupled with bromelain, which is an extract of pineapple. Take supplements on an empty stomach.	150–450 mg three times a day
Nettle	Nettle is a well-known folk remedy used for hay fever and other allergies. It can help clear congestion and relieve inflammation.	300 mg three times a day
Eyebright	Eyebright is an herb that can be effective in relieving the symptoms of hay fever, especially itchy and streaming eyes.	2–6 ml of tincture three times a day

4

ASTHMA

Asthma is a chronic lung condition characterized by recurrent attacks of breathlessness, often accompanied by wheezing. Asthma is due to inflammation in the air passages in the lungs, causing constriction of these passages (bronchospasm), which makes breathing difficult. Asthma can be classified into two main types: extrinsic, in which attacks are triggered by an allergy, and intrinsic, in which there is no obvious external cause. Extrinsic or "allergic" asthma tends to come on during childhood, while intrinsic asthma usually develops later in life. However, either condition can appear at any age.

ASTHMA TRIGGERS

Allergic asthma is often set off by an inhaled trigger substance such as animal fur, dust, feathers, or air pollutants. However, there is also good evidence that asthma attacks can be linked to certain foods, particularly in childhood asthma. Probably the most common offenders in this respect are dairy products based on cow's milk. Child asthmatics often find significant relief by eliminating cow's milk, cheese, and yogurt, and replacing them with soy and rice milk, goat's cheese, and soy, goat's, and sheep's yogurt.

4

ASTHMA AND EXERCISE

In years gone by, it used to be assumed that children who suffered from asthma needed to avoid strenuous exercise for fear of bringing on an attack of breathlessness. Nowadays, asthma can be effectively controlled by medical treatments supported by natural measures, so in most cases an asthmatic child can enjoy the full range of activities and need not be restricted to a sedentary life.

HIDDEN EXTRAS

Children with asthma can be sensitive to food additives such as artificial sweeteners, colorings, preservatives, and flavorings. Eliminating processed foods with artificial additives can bring about a significant improvement in some children.

There is quite a lot of evidence, too, linking salt consumption with asthma. Salt appears to heighten the airways' response to histamine, causing increased constriction. Asthmatics should therefore avoid adding salt to their food during cooking or at the table, and minimize their consumption of processed foods, which tend to have a lot of salt already added.

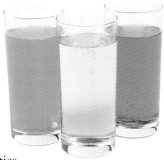
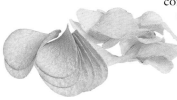

USEFUL SUPPLEMENTS

Supplement	Action	Dose
Quercetin	Studies have shown that quercetin is an antihistamine and can therefore block allergic reactions. It also has anti-inflammatory properties that may reduce irritation in the lining of the airways.	500 mg twice a day
Bromelain	This extract of pineapple has potent anti-inflammatory activity in the body and can also enhance the effectiveness of quercetin when taken in combination with it.	500 mg twice a day
Vitamin C	Vitamin C is another natural antihistamine that may help reduce allergic attacks in asthma. Women taking oral contraceptives should take a maximum daily dose of no more than 1000 mg.	1000 mg three times a day
Ginkgo biloba	Ginkgo biloba contains several unique substances known collectively as ginkgolides that block the effect of a key chemical in the processes that trigger asthma.	40 mg of standardized extract three times a day

4

EAR INFECTIONS

Middle ear infections (also called "otitis media" by the medical profession) are common in childhood and a frequent cause of earache. Such infections are quite often related to colds when the viral infection may lead to the buildup of fluid and congestion, making infection with a bacterial agent more likely. Bacterial infections are usually treated with antibiotics.

FOOD SENSITIVITY

In natural medicine it is often found that recurrent middle-ear infections in children are related to sensitivity to particular foods. Children who were breastfed are less likely to suffer from this kind of problem than those who were bottle-fed. Some foods are renowned for their ability to stimulate mucus formation in and around the ears, with dairy products being by far the most common culprits.

ELIMINATING TRIGGERS

If your child suffers from repeated ear infections, substitute rice and soy milk (available from health food stores), and cheeses made from goat's and sheep's milk for cow's milk and dairy products made from cow's milk. If your child does not improve on this regime, you might try eliminating other commonly implicated foods such as wheat, eggs, and chocolate. Sugar should also be avoided since it suppresses immune function.

4

MIDDLE EAR FLUID

Otitis media, or middle ear fluid, is a condition characterized by the buildup of fluid behind the ear drum and affects about 30 percent of children under the age of six. The condition usually causes hearing problems and increases the likelihood of earache and infection. The conventional medical approach to glue ear is to insert tiny plastic tubes into the ear drum. This allows air into the middle ear, enabling excess fluid to drain from this area. The condition is often found to be the result of one or more food sensitivities, so following the same food exclusion advice as for ear infections may help control a child's symptoms.

USEFUL SUPPLEMENTS

The additional supplements recommended for preventing and treating colds and flu are also useful for ear infections.

Supplement	Action	Dose
Echinacea	This herb can help improve immune efficiency and may help to clear ear infections. Use a supplement specifically designed for children or adjust the dose of the supplement according to body weight.	Follow the instructions on the label
Acidophilus	Children who have had an ear infection will normally have been given antibiotics. While these may help fight bacterial infection in the ear itself, they can also kill many of the beneficial bacteria in the gut leading to imbalance in the organisms here. This, in the long term, may lead to other problems including irritable bowel syndrome and food sensitivities. Preparations of one of the intestinal tract's most important organisms – acidophilus – will help to restore the balance of organisms in a child's gut. Such supplements can be bought in powder form or as capsules that can be opened and taken in water.	1–10 billion live organisms a day
Zinc	Zinc supplementation can increase immune function and may help to prevent recurrence of ear infections. Adjust the dose to the weight of your child.	5 mg of zinc per day (for a child weighing 30 lb/15 kg)
Vitamin A	Vitamin A is required by the immune system and may help recovery from ear infection. Give supplements while your child's symptoms persist.	5000 IU per day (child's dose)

4

URINE INFECTIONS

Infections of the urinary tract, including cystitis and urethritis, are usually caused by the overgrowth of bacteria in the urine. Common symptoms include low abdominal discomfort, frequent urination, and a burning or stinging sensation on passing water. Anyone suffering from persistent symptoms should see his or her doctor in case treatment with antibiotics is necessary.

PREVENTING INFECTION

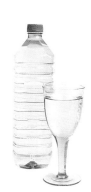

It may be possible to protect yourself from further infections through certain lifestyle changes and the use of specific nutritional supplements. Be sure to drink plenty of filtered or spring water each day, which will help to wash out any unhealthy germs before they get the opportunity to multiply in the bladder. Bacteria can often be introduced into the urinary tract during sexual intercourse. Passing water as soon as possible after sex will help to flush out germs that may be making their way toward the bladder.

DIETARY MEASURES

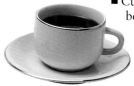

4

■ Cut your sugar and alcohol consumption to a minimum because both of these inhibit the immune system and make it less likely that you will clear the infection naturally.

■ Coffee and citrus fruits tend to irritate the bladder, so avoid these, too.

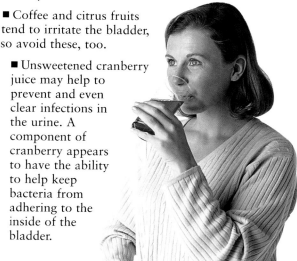

■ Unsweetened cranberry juice may help to prevent and even clear infections in the urine. A component of cranberry appears to have the ability to help keep bacteria from adhering to the inside of the bladder.

BARLEY WATER

Barley water is a traditional remedy for urinary-tract infections. It is made by boiling a teaspoon of barley in one quart of water for an hour. Strain and flavor the water with lemon juice and honey. Drink as required.

GENERAL HYGIENE

Personal hygiene is important for preventing urinary-tract infections.

■ Women and girls should always wipe from front to back after going to the toilet.

■ Change underwear daily.

■ Avoid using fragranced products, such as soaps or deodorants, in the genital area.

USEFUL SUPPLEMENTS

Supplement	Action	Dose
Cranberry extract	Cranberry extract can help prevent and treat infections through its ability to inhibit the bacterial colonization of the bladder. Cranberry also contains substances known as anthocyanosides, which are natural antibiotics and may help to keep bacteria under control.	400 mg of extract twice a day
Uva ursi	This herb has been used for more than 1,000 years by the Chinese and Native Americans to treat urinary-tract infections. The herb contains a substance called arbutin, which is converted in the urine to hydroquinone, a urinary antiseptic. Uva ursi is also a natural diuretic, helping to flush out the kidneys. Avoid if you are pregnant or breastfeeding.	250–500 mg of extract, three times a day for a total of 14 days
Acidophilus	Women who suffer from recurrent bouts of cystitis may often take antibiotics to control infections. Antibiotics may kill many of the beneficial bacteria in the gut, leading to imbalance in the organisms here. It is believed that such an imbalance may contribute to vaginal yeast infections (candida), which in turn may make problems with cystitis more likely. Taking an acidophilus supplement may help prevent recurrent urinary-tract infections in the long term.	1–10 billion live organisms a day

4

CANCER PREVENTION

The cells in the body are constantly being renewed and replaced. As old, worn-out cells die, younger cells divide to replace them. This process usually goes on in an orderly, controlled fashion. However, sometimes a cell can begin dividing much more quickly than it should, leading to the formation of a cancerous tumor.

CANCER AND DIET

Up to 70 percent of cancers are related to diet. For instance, a large amount of fat in the diet is linked with an increased risk of cancer. This seems to apply particularly to cancers of the breast, colon, rectum, ovary, and prostate. The precise role of fat in cancer is not yet known, although some evidence exists to suggest that fats in the blood are important for the growth of certain tumors.

DIETARY CARCINOGENS

Eating large amounts of salt-cured, salt-pickled, and smoked foods has been linked to cancer of the esophagus. The smoke from curing seems to create cancer-promoting agents called carcinogens in the food, while salt-cured and salt-pickled foods contain chemicals that can be converted into carcinogens in the food or in the stomach. Grilling or barbecuing food over an open flame can also create carcinogens on the surface of foods, particularly if the food is charred and fatty.

ALCOHOL AND SMOKING

4

The consumption of alcohol appears to increase the risk of developing certain forms of cancer. In moderate amounts, alcohol seems to be linked to an increased risk of cancers of the breast, rectum, and pancreas. In excessive amounts, especially when combined with cigarette smoking, alcohol may also increase the likelihood of cancer of the mouth, esophagus, and larynx.

FREE RADICALS

The process that triggers cancer in the body is thought to be related to the production of damaging, destructive molecules in the body called free radicals. Free radicals are neutralized by the antioxidant nutrients such as vitamins A, C, and E and the mineral selenium. The best diet to help prevent cancer is therefore a low-fat, high-fiber diet, containing plenty of foods rich in antioxidant nutrients. A diet rich in fresh fruits, vegetables, and whole grains like whole-wheat bread and brown rice fulfills all these criteria.

USEFUL SUPPLEMENTS

Supplement	Action	Dose
Vitamin A	Vitamin A appears to have an important role to play in keeping the body free from cancer. Low levels are associated with an increased risk of cancers of the lung, throat, esophagus (gullet), mouth, stomach, colon, and prostate. Do not take more than 10,000 IU a day if you are pregnant or planning pregnancy.	5,000–10,000 IU a day
Betacarotene	Betacarotene is converted into vitamin A in the body, but is thought to have some cancer-protecting qualities of its own.	25,000–50,000 IU a day
Vitamin C	Vitamin C is a potent antioxidant and powerful immune stimulant. An enormous body of evidence exists linking high intakes of vitamin C with enhanced protection from cancer, particularly cancers of the lung, rectum, esophagus, mouth, stomach, and pancreas. Women taking oral contraceptives should take no more than 1000 mg a day.	2–4 g a day
Vitamin E	Vitamin E is an important antioxidant, and also can deactivate some cancer-causing chemicals in the body. Low levels of vitamin E are associated with an increased risk of cancer, particularly of the esophagus and stomach. Its anticancer properties appear to be most evident when it is coupled with selenium.	400 IU a day
Selenium	Selenium is a trace mineral that has an important cancer-protecting role in the body. Individuals with low levels of selenium in their blood have three times the risk of cancer than those with higher levels. One study found that 200 mcg of selenium each day halved the risk of cancer. Selenium exerts its beneficial effect in the body in combination with vitamin E.	200 mcg a day

4

HIV AND AIDS

Infection with the HIV organism can compromise the healthy function of the immune system and eventually lead to AIDS. Reduced immune function leads to increased susceptibility to a wide range of infections, and increased risk of certain cancers. Nutritional deficiencies can further impair immune function, increasing the risk of complications. Many of those infected by HIV can improve their general health and resistance to infection by adjustments to their diet and by taking nutritional supplements in consultation with their medical advisers.

IMMUNITY-BOOSTING FOODS

The diet should be based on nutrient-rich foods such as fresh fruits, vegetables, and whole grains. Protein malnutrition is quite common in AIDS, so beans, legumes, tofu, and fish should be included in the diet. Sugar should be avoided since it tends to disable the immune system.

USEFUL SUPPLEMENTS

Supplement	Action	Dose
Multivitamin and mineral preparation	Take a good-quality, high-potency multivitamin and mineral supplement to correct and prevent any nutritional deficiencies.	Follow the instructions on the label
Vitamin C	Vitamin C is a potent immune enhancer and also has antiviral activity.	3000–5000 mg a day
Zinc	This mineral is essential for the function of the immune system.	30–45 mg a day
Coenzyme Q10	Coenzyme Q10 is responsible for the manufacture of ATP, which is the essential currency used for energy production in each cell in the body. Supplementing with this nutrient can improve energy levels and enhances antioxidant activity in the body.	30 mg three times a day

4

Blood, Hormones, and Metabolism

5

BLOOD, HORMONES, AND METABOLISM

The blood and the circulation are responsible for carrying oxygen and nutrients to every tissue. Without an adequate blood supply, tissues and organs are unable to operate efficiently. The circulation of blood in the body is dependent on a strong heart and a healthy network of vessels through which the blood is pumped.

Changes in the constituents of the blood can sometimes lead to illness, too. For instance, a failure of the body to make enough red blood cells may lead to anemia. This chapter looks at natural approaches to preventing and combating disorders of blood circulation including heart disease, high blood pressure, and poor circulation, as well as problems of blood composition.

5

ANEMIA

Oxygen is transported throughout the body by red blood cells. The substance in the red blood cells responsible for carrying oxygen is called hemoglobin. Anemia is a condition where there is a shortage of red blood cells or hemoglobin or both. In anemia, the body's tissues are starved of oxygen, which usually causes physical and mental fatigue. Sufferers may also have a pale complexion.

THE CAUSES OF ANEMIA

Anemia can be related to deficiencies of several different nutrients, including iron, folic acid, and vitamin B_{12}. A blood test will help determine which form of anemia you are suffering from. In addition, your doctor may want to investigate the underlying cause of your anemia. Of all the potential causes of anemia, iron deficiency is the most common. If you are suffering from iron-deficiency anemia, make sure you eat plenty of foods rich in iron. Iron-rich foods include:

- Broccoli, greens, and cabbage.

- Almonds.

- Eggs.

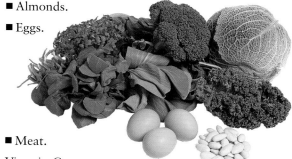

- Meat.

Vitamin C can enhance the absorption of iron, so it is also important to eat plenty of vitamin C-rich foods such as fresh fruits and vegetables.

Warning

While anemia is a common cause of fatigue, it is not a problem that should be self-diagnosed. Before treatment for anemia can be started, the diagnosis should be confirmed with a blood test. Your doctor will be able to do this for you.

5

PERNICIOUS ANEMIA

Pernicious anemia is a particular sort of anemia caused by a chronic deficiency of vitamin B_{12}. Sufferers of this condition lack the ability to make a molecule in the stomach called "intrinsic factor," which is necessary if B_{12} is to be absorbed properly by the body. As a result, dietary sources of B_{12}, even in supplement form, are not absorbed. People who have pernicious anemia therefore require regular B_{12} injections to prevent deficiency.

OTHER ESSENTIAL NUTRIENTS

Apart from iron, the other essential blood nutrients are folic acid and vitamin B_{12} (also known as cobalamin). Folic acid can be found in green leafy vegetables and whole grains such as whole-wheat bread and whole-wheat pasta. B_{12} is primarily found in animal products, including meat, fish, eggs, and dairy foods. For this reason, B_{12} deficiency is more common in vegans than in the general population. If your diet does not contain animal products, you are very likely to have some degree of B_{12} deficiency and would be well advised to take a regular supplement.

USEFUL SUPPLEMENTS

Supplement	Action	Dose
Iron	Iron is essential for the production of hemoglobin, which is the pigment in red blood cells that carries oxygen.	50–100 mg daily with food
Vitamin C	Vitamin C enhances the absorption of iron.	500–1000 mg taken with iron
Folic acid	Folic acid is necessary for cells to divide normally. Deficiency of this nutrient may therefore lead to anemia by hampering the division of red blood cells.	400 mcg a day
Vitamin B_{12}	B_{12} works with folic acid in many body processes, including the manufacture of new red blood cells.	800–1000 mcg a day

5

POOR CIRCULATION

Cold hands and feet are usually caused by a constriction of the small vessels that take blood into the fingers and toes. Sometimes excessive narrowing of these small blood vessels in the skin leads to the development of chilblains. These itchy, purple-red swellings, which usually occur on the fingers or toes, can be quite uncomfortable but are not serious. Chilblains occur mostly in the young and the elderly, and are more common in women than in men. In conventional medicine the usual advice for those with circulatory problems is to invest in some thermal socks and gloves. Natural medicine, however, offers other strategies that may improve circulation and therefore relieve coldness of the hands and feet.

HEALTHY AND UNHEALTHY FATS

For healthy circulation it is important to avoid the types of fats found in red meat, dairy products, and fried and processed foods. Regular consumption of these fats causes narrowing of blood vessels. Healthy fats such as extra-virgin olive oil, and the oils derived from seeds and found in oily fish, such as salmon, trout, mackerel, and herring, seem to improve circulation in the long term, so make sure you include plenty of them in your diet. Also, avoid caffeine, which generally leads to constriction of blood vessels.

USEFUL SUPPLEMENTS		
Supplement	**Action**	**Dose**
Fish oil	Fish oil helps prevent further buildup of fat on the artery walls and may reduce spasm in the vessels.	I g three times a day
Vitamin E	These nutrients help to improve blood flow and may reduce constriction of the blood vessels.	400 IU a day
Ginkgo biloba	This herb is known for its ability to enhance the circulation. Not only can it improve blood flow to the hands and feet, but it may also enhance blood supply to the brain, thereby improving memory.	40 mg of standardized extract three times a day

5

VARICOSE VEINS

Veins transport blood from the body's tissues back to the heart. Each vein contains valves that keep blood flowing toward the heart and prevent it from going in the other direction. If the wall of the vein or the valves within it become weakened, blood may pool in the vein, causing it to become dilated. This is commonly referred to as a varicose vein. Varicose veins can tend to run in families, but may also be related to other factors such as pregnancy and prolonged periods of sitting or standing. Varicose veins affect about half the adult population to some degree, but are four times more common in women than in men.

KEEP WALKING

Exercise may help to prevent varicose vein formation, because it helps to circulate blood around the body. A good brisk walk for half an hour or so a day may well help stop varicose veins from developing any further.

USEFUL SUPPLEMENTS

Supplement	Action	Dose
Grape seed extract	This substance contains oligomeric procyanidins (OPCs), which have the ability to strengthen blood vessel walls and may therefore help shrink and even eliminate varicose veins.	150–300 mg a day
Vitamin E	Vitamin E can help reduce the severity of varicose veins, perhaps by improving circulation in the legs. The dose of vitamin E should be increased gradually in anyone with a history of high blood pressure.	400 IU a day
Butcher's broom	Rustrogenis, the active ingredient of this herb, can help to reduce the discomfort caused by varicose veins.	50–100 mg of extract a day

5

HIGH CHOLESTEROL

Cholesterol is a waxy, fatlike substance that is transported around the body in the bloodstream. Cholesterol can build up on the inside of our arteries and increase our risk of cardiovascular diseases such as heart disease and stroke. The deposition of cholesterol in artery walls is known as "atherosclerosis." Generally, the higher the level of cholesterol in the blood, the greater the risk of atherosclerosis.

REDUCING FAT INTAKE

Anyone who is suffering from a higher-than-normal level of cholesterol in their blood should cut down on his or her consumption of fat, especially red meat, dairy products, and fried and processed foods. However, while some fats seem to raise cholesterol levels, others have a more beneficial effect.

FOODS THAT LOWER CHOLESTEROL

Extra-virgin olive oil and the fats found in oily fish such as salmon, mackerel, and trout are generally beneficial to health and may actually help to lower cholesterol levels. A high-fiber diet can also help reduce cholesterol levels in the blood, possibly by binding to fat in the gut and preventing its absorption into the body. For this reason, a good diet should be rich in fruits, vegetables, beans, and legumes.

CHOLESTEROL AND THE LIVER

Most of the cholesterol in the body does not come from the diet, but is manufactured naturally in the liver. This is why dietary changes sometimes seem to have relatively little impact on a raised cholesterol level.

5

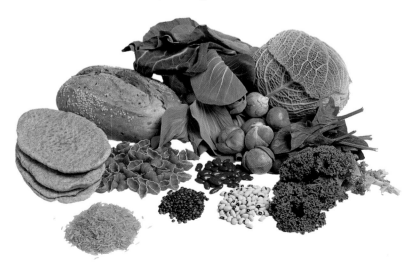

THE ROLE OF TRIGLYCERIDES

Fat is transported around the body in two main forms – cholesterol and triglycerides. Triglycerides are the major form of fat found in food and the body. While the precise impact of triglycerides on health is unclear, there is evidence linking high levels of triglycerides in the blood with an increased risk of heart disease. Triglyceride levels can be raised by consuming sugar, so it is important to reduce consumption of all sugary foods and drink. Alcohol in excess can also increase triglyceride levels. The supplements that may help to reduce triglycerides in the blood are the same as those that may combat raised cholesterol levels.

CALCULATING ALCOHOL INTAKE

Aim to drink no more than one or two units a day – a unit is equivalent to a small glass of wine, a small measure of hard liquor, or ½ pint (25 cl) of beer.

Each of these drinks contains
one unit of alcohol

 = =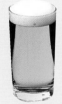

| I small glass of wine | I small measure of hard liquor | I small glass of beer |

USEFUL SUPPLEMENTS

Supplement	Action	Dose
Fish oil	Fish oil supplements rich in essential fats eicosapentaenoic (EPA) and docosahexanoic acid (DHA) have a positive effect on the heart and circulation. High consumption of fish oils is thought to explain why the Inuit peoples of North America enjoy an extremely low incidence of heart disease.	I g three times a day
Chromium	This trace mineral can help reduce cholesterol levels in the blood.	200–400 mcg a day
Garlic	Garlic helps to reduce cholesterol levels in the blood and is thought to have a number of other important beneficial effects on the heart and circulation.	500 mg of garlic extract a day

5

HIGH BLOOD PRESSURE

High blood pressure (often referred to as hypertension by doctors) is a very common problem, and affects about one in seven of the adult population. Although it usually produces no symptoms itself, it does substantially increase our risk of cardiovascular problems such as stroke and heart attack.

THE CAUSES OF HIGH BLOOD PRESSURE

High blood pressure is usually closely related to certain lifestyle factors. For instance, smoking and obesity can substantially increase the risk of suffering from high blood pressure. If you smoke, you should stop or at least cut down. If you are overweight or obese, you will almost certainly benefit from losing some of the excess weight. The link between stress and high blood pressure is less clearly established. However, learning how to handle stress in your life can benefit many other aspects of your health.

MEASURING BLOOD PRESSURE

Blood pressure is the pressure, or tension, of the blood within the arteries of the circulatory system. Your blood pressure is expressed as two values, one over the other e.g. 120/70. The upper value refers to the systolic pressure, which is the maximum pressure that occurs during contraction of the heart. The lower value, or diastolic pressure, is the minimum pressure during the resting period of the heart. Generally, blood pressure of less than 130/80 is regarded as healthy. Blood pressure of 140/90 or more is considered to be high. Blood pressures between 130/85 and 140/90 are generally classified as "borderline high." Individuals in this category may not receive treatment immediately.

Systolic	mmHg	Diastolic
	160	
	155	
	150	
	145	
High	140	
	135	
Borderline high	130	
Healthy	125	
	120	
	115	
	110	
	105	
	100	
	95	
	90	High
	85	Borderline high
	80	Healthy
	75	
	70	

5

LOWERING BLOOD PRESSURE

In the long term, this is best achieved by eating a healthful diet in conjunction with a sensible exercise regimen.

■ Salt appears to have a very important effect on blood pressure, too. Do not add salt during cooking or at the table, and avoid processed and packaged foods that tend to have a lot of salt already added.

■ Lose weight if you are overweight. Cut down on sugary and fatty foods while increasing your intake of fruits, vegetables, and whole grains.

■ Exercise has also been shown to reduce blood pressure directly. Try to take some form of exercise (brisk walking is ideal) for half an hour every day. If you are unused to strenuous exercise, check with your doctor first.

■ Do not smoke. Substances in tobacco smoke tend to raise blood pressure.

■ Moderate your alcohol intake. Do not drink more than two units (see page 85) a day.

USEFUL SUPPLEMENTS

Supplement	Action	Dose
Fish oil	Fish oil has been shown to have a beneficial effect on the lining of our body's vessels and may help reduce blood pressure.	I g three times a day
Calcium	There are many studies that exist which show that calcium may help lower blood pressure. Calcium supplementation appears to have the effect of preventing high blood pressure, too.	1000 mg a day
Magnesium	Magnesium may help reduce blood pressure, probably through its ability to relax the muscles present in the walls of the major arteries in the body.	500 mg a day
Hawthorn	Studies on humans and animals have shown that this herb can lower blood pressure during exertion and may strengthen the heart's ability to pump blood. Hawthorn is also a natural diuretic that helps the body rid itself of excess salt and water.	80–300 mg of extract three times a day

5

HEART DISEASE

The heart muscle is supplied with oxygen and nutrients via three vessels that can be seen on the surface of the heart called the coronary arteries. As we age, the coronary arteries can become clogged with a fatlike substance called atheroma, giving rise to a condition known as ischemic heart disease (IHD). Should one or more vessels block off completely, part of the heart muscle may die. This is commonly referred to as a heart attack.

KEY DIET ADVICE

Anyone suffering from heart disease or who is keen to prevent it should eat a diet low in saturated (animal) fat and sugar but high in fresh fruits and vegetables. Some foods, principally extra-virgin olive oil and oily fish, seem to give positive protection against heart disease and should be included in the diet. Substitute fish for meat and cook with good-quality olive oil rather than butter or margarine.

ARRHYTHMIAS

The heart has its own electrical circuitry that is responsible for keeping it beating regularly, about 60 to 70 times each minute. Sometimes, the heart's circuitry can misfire, producing fast, slow, weakened, or irregular contractions. Common symptoms during an attack include palpitations, breathlessness, fatigue, and lightheadedness. If you have problems of heart rhythm, there are several practical measures you can take:

■ Avoid alcohol and caffeine, both of which tend to disrupt the normal rhythm of the heart.

■ Avoid foods that contain cayenne or chili pepper because these seem to have a stimulating effect on the heart.

■ Make sure you eat plenty of foods rich in magnesium and potassium. These nutrients are very important in keeping the heart beating properly. Nuts, seafood, seeds, green leafy vegetables, and whole grains such as whole-wheat bread and whole-wheat pasta are rich in magnesium, while potassium can be found in fresh fruits and vegetables, especially bananas.

5

THE ROLE OF EXERCISE

Exercise is vital to the health of the heart. However, it is important that you start slowly and build up as your fitness level increases. To begin with, take half an hour of gentle exercise three or four times a week. Anyone with a history of heart disease should consult a doctor before embarking on any exercise regimen.

USEFUL SUPPLEMENTS

Supplement	Action	Dose
Magnesium	Magnesium is essential for the healthy conduction of nerve signals though the heart muscle.	250 mg twice a day
Coenzyme Q10	This supplement may help to regulate heart rhythm.	30 mg two or three times a day
Vitamin E	Vitamin E may be an effective treatment for heart disease. It is also an effective preventive agent and has been shown to reduce the risk of heart disease by about 40 percent in the long term. If there is any history of high blood pressure, vitamin E should be started at a dose of 100 IU a day and gradually increased over a few weeks. This should be done in consultation with your doctor.	100–200 IU a day
Fish oil	Fish oil has a blood-thinning effect and helps prevent fatty buildup in the arteries.	1 g three times a day
Garlic	Garlic is well known to have a broad range of beneficial effects on the cardiovascular system.	500 mg of garlic extract each day

5

DIABETES

Sugar levels in the bloodstream are regulated by several hormones, the most important of which is insulin. The effect of insulin in the body is to keep blood sugar levels in check. If this mechanism fails, the blood sugar level rises and diabetes is the result. In the long term, diabetes can lead to a variety of health problems including eye disease and blindness, kidney disease, heart disease, leg ulcers, gangrene, and impotence.

TYPES OF DIABETES

There are essentially two forms of diabetes – Type 1 and Type 2. Type 1 diabetes (also known as juvenile onset or insulin-dependent diabetes) comes on early in life and is caused by a failure of the pancreas to secrete insulin. Sufferers from this form of diabetes must take insulin by injection to keep blood sugar levels from rising uncontrollably.

Type 2 diabetes (also known as mature onset or non-insulin dependent diabetes) usually comes on in middle or old age. Here, often the problem is not that there is insufficient insulin, but the body is resistant to its effects. People with this form of diabetes may be able to control their diabetes through changing their diet. If this fails, oral medication may be prescribed, and a proportion of Type 2 people with diabetes eventually need insulin to control their condition.

Warning

People with diabetes should consult their doctor before making any dietary changes or altering the prescribed dose of medication .

SLOW-RELEASE SUGAR

For all people with diabetes it is important to avoid foods that release sugar quickly into the bloodstream. High sugar foods such as soft drinks, candy, chocolate, sugared breakfast cereals, cookies, and cakes cause the level of sugar in the bloodstream to rise rapidly, disrupting blood sugar balance. Other foods that tend to release sugar quickly include potatoes, white bread, white rice, and white pasta. These should therefore be avoided or eaten in moderation. Your diet should be based around foods that release sugar slowly into the bloodstream, such as unrefined carbohydrates and vegetables (other than potatoes), and those that help to slow sugar release from other foods. Such foods include meat and fish.

5

BLOOD SUGAR LEVELS AFTER EATING

People with diabetes need to keep blood sugar levels as stable as possible. People with non-insulin dependent diabetes can often reduce their need for drugs by basing the diet around foods that release their energy slowly into the bloodstream, and therefore stimulate gradual release of insulin which keeps levels of sugar in the blood within healthy limits. If foods are eaten that release large amounts of sugar into the bloodstream rapidly, excess sugar is likely to remain in the bloodstream longer.

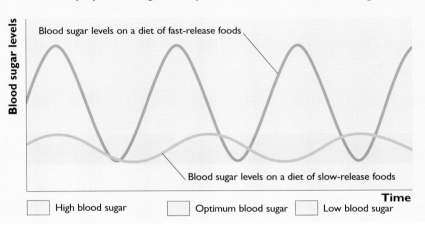

USEFUL SUPPLEMENTS

Supplement	Action	Dose
Chromium	Studies show that this nutrient can improve blood sugar control. Avoid in pregnancy.	200–400 mcg a day
Gymnema sylvestre	The leaves of the gymnema sylvestre plant, which grows in the tropical forests of central and southern India, have been employed in the treatment of diabetes for many centuries. Studies demonstrate that the herb may help reduce blood sugar levels in both insulin-dependent and non-insulin dependent diabetes. In a proportion of people with diabetes the requirement for medication is significantly reduced, and some on oral medication may be able to stop taking their medication completely.	400 mg a day

5

PROSTATE DISEASE

The prostate is a walnut-sized gland that surrounds the first part of the urethra, the tube that takes urine from the bladder to the outside. As a man ages, the prostate gland may enlarge, which can impede the flow of urine from the bladder.

ENLARGED PROSTATE

Typical symptoms of prostatic enlargement include poor urinary stream, frequent urination, difficulty starting urination, dribbling after urination, and the need to get up at night to pass water. Prostate enlargement is normally due to a condition called benign prostatic hyperplasia (BPH), which is a common condition after the age of 50.

PROSTATIC CANCER

While benign prostatic hyperplasia is the most common cause of prostate enlargement, it is not the only condition to affect this gland. The prostate can be affected by cancer, and anyone who has the symptoms of prostate enlargement should see their doctor for a proper assessment. Prostatic cancer is one of the most common male conditions and is the second most common cancer in men. However, it is usually a slow-growing cancer, and most sufferers die of an unrelated illness.

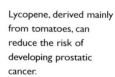

Lycopene, derived mainly from tomatoes, can reduce the risk of developing prostatic cancer.

THE EFFECTS OF SOY

The rate of prostate cancer in Japan is much lower than it is in the West. It is thought that this difference may be related to the higher consumption of soy-based foods such as tofu in Japan. Soybean contains substances called isoflavones, which appear to have the ability to block the effect of the hormones that are thought to play a part in triggering prostate cancer. Isoflavones can be taken as a supplement. The recommended dose is 40 mg per day. An equivalent amount can be obtained from a cup of soy milk or 3–4 oz (80 to 100 g) of tofu.

5

USEFUL SUPPLEMENTS

Nutritional supplements and herbal remedies have produced beneficial effects in treating enlargement of the prostate and reducing the risk of prostatic cancer.

Supplement	Action	Dose
Lycopene	This relative of betacarotene is obtained mainly from tomatoes. A high intake seems to reduce the risk of developing prostatic cancer.	10 mg a day
Selenium	One study has shown that 200 mcg of selenium each day can reduce the risk of developing prostatic cancer by about 67 percent.	200 mcg a day
Saw palmetto	This herb has a long history of use by Native Americans. Researchers believe that Saw palmetto works by deactivating an enzyme in the body that is involved in the conversion of testosterone to a more potent version of this hormone called dihydrotestosterone. Dihydrotestosterone has the ability to stimulate prostatic cell growth, so blocking its production can lead to a reduction in prostate size. Saw palmetto is effective in relieving symptoms in the majority of sufferers.	160 mg twice a day
African pygeum	African pygeum is a large evergreen tree, the bark of which is used to produce the herbal extract. The herb contains compounds that block the production of hormonelike substances called prostaglandins – these play an important part in inflammation, particularly in the prostate.	50–100 mg of standardized extract twice a day
Linseed oil	There are many anecdotal reports that linseed oil can help reduce symptoms of prostate enlargement.	1 g two or three times a day
Zinc	This mineral is found in very high concentration in the prostate and is thought to play an important role in its health.	15–45 mg a day

5

GALLSTONES

The gallbladder is a saclike structure that lies underneath and is attached to the liver. The liver makes a substance called bile which passes to and is then concentrated in the gallbladder. When a fatty meal is eaten, the gallbladder contracts, squirting bile down a tube called the bile duct, which is in turn connected to the first part of the small bowel (duodenum). Bile acts in the digestive tract to emulsify fat, effectively dissolving it into tiny droplets that can then be fully broken down by fat-digesting enzymes. Sometimes, hard stones known as gallstones may form in the gallbladder. These are often composed of solidified cholesterol and are more likely to occur in people who are overweight.

SYMPTOMS

Most people with gallstones have no symptoms and are unaware that they even have them. However, in about 20 percent of cases, the gallstones do cause problems, with pain under the ribs on the right side and indigestion made worse by fatty foods being the most common symptoms.

GALLSTONE TREATMENTS

Depending on the type of gallstones, drugs may sometimes be prescribed to shrink them. In some cases, ultrasound waves may be used to shatter the stones, which then pass out of the gallbladder into the bowel. Nonsurgical treatments are safe, but may not prevent the recurrence of stones. A significant proportion of sufferers eventually come to have their gallbladder removed surgically, a procedure that doctors call "cholecystectomy."

FOODS TO AVOID

To help prevent cholesterol gallstones from forming, and also to reduce your risk of symptoms, make the following changes to your diet:

■ Reduce the amount of saturated fat in your diet to a minimum by cutting back on red meat, dairy products, and fried and processed foods.

■ Avoid onions, eggs, and chocolate, which all quite commonly trigger attacks of pain.

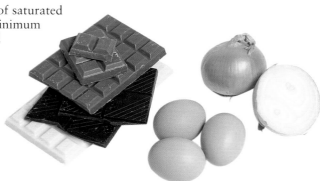

5

Warning

If pain from suspected gallstones persists for more than a few hours or becomes severe, seek immediate medical advice.

BENEFICIAL FOODS

Your diet should be based on whole, unprocessed foods such as whole-wheat bread, brown rice, beans, fruits, and vegetables, because eating a high-fiber diet can reduce the risk of gallstones in the long term. This type of diet will also help you lose excess weight if you need to.

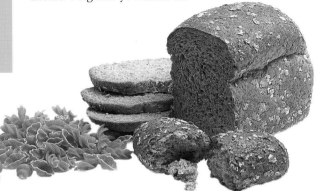

USEFUL SUPPLEMENTS

Supplement	Action	Dose
Lecithin	Lecithin is a phospholipid, a class of compounds produced by the liver which are involved in the metabolism of fat. This common constituent of animal and plant tissues is a natural source of choline, which can help prevent gallstone formation. Take a tablespoon of lecithin granules twice a day, dissolved in some water or fruit juice.	350–500 mg (products containing 90 percent phosphatidyl-choline)
Milk thistle	This herb has a variety of positive effects on the liver, the health of which is critical to proper gallbladder function. It is thought that one effect of milk thistle is to increase the solubility of bile, preventing stagnation of bile and thereby reducing the likelihood of the formation of gallstones.	100–150 mg three times a day

5

KIDNEY STONES

Kidney stones come in several different forms, the most common of which are made of calcium and a substance called oxalate. Because it is generally believed that a diet rich in calcium could predispose to stone formation, sufferers are often advised to cut down on their intake of this mineral. However, an American study showed that individuals who eat a calcium-rich diet were actually less likely to get kidney stones than those who eat a diet low in calcium. If anything, it is a high level of oxalate in the diet that seems to predispose to the most common form of kidney stone.

WHAT YOU CAN DO

If you have kidney stones, cut down on your consumption of oxalate-rich foods. Common examples include:

- Beets and spinach.
- Strawberries, rhubarb, and gooseberries.
- Nuts and chocolate.
- Tea.

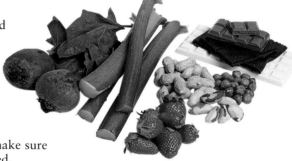

In addition, make sure you drink at least six to eight glasses of filtered or spring water every day to make sure your kidneys are well flushed.

5

USEFUL SUPPLEMENTS

Supplement	Action	Dose
Potassium	Potassium may help prevent the buildup of stones.	100 mg twice a day
Magnesium	This mineral may help to dissolve small stones before they become a problem.	500 mg a day
Vitamin B$_6$	May help to dissolve small stones.	50 mg twice a day

Women's Health and Pregnancy

6

WOMEN'S HEALTH AND PREGNANCY

Menstruation, menopause, and pregnancy are a natural part of womanhood, but may also bring problems. Vitamins, minerals, and herbs can be very effective in restoring hormonal balance to a woman's body, thereby relieving many of the symptoms of the female-specific conditions. There is growing evidence that the nutritional status of a mother can have an important influence on her pregnancy and the health of her child. This chapter gives advice on which supplements may benefit pregnancy and help relieve pregnancy-related conditions such as morning sickness.

6

PERIOD PROBLEMS

The body of the uterus is made up of muscular tissue. During a menstrual period, this muscle contracts to help expel the lining of the uterus. Sometimes, the contractions can be very strong, and this can lead to severe discomfort, the medical term for which is dysmenorrhea. For some women blood loss may also be excessively heavy, a problem known as menorrhagia.

SYMPTOMS AND CAUSES OF PAIN

Dysmenorrhea is typically felt as a cramplike pain or discomfort in the lower abdomen, which may come and go in waves. Backache is a common accompanying symptom. Dysmenorrhea is thought to be related to hormonal changes during a period. One theory is that the pain is caused by excessive production of or sensitivity to hormonelike substances called prostaglandins. These are thought to stimulate muscular spasm in the uterus.

REDUCING CRAMPS

The nutrients calcium and magnesium are essential to muscle function, and can be very effective in reducing menstrual cramps. Increase your consumption of foods rich in these nutrients including sardines, mackerel, and green leafy vegetables. Nutrients to treat dysmenorrhea should ideally be started several days before your period is expected.

USEFUL SUPPLEMENTS FOR PAINFUL PERIODS

Supplement	Action	Dose
Calcium and magnesium	Additional quantities of calcium and magnesium in supplement form can be very effective in relieving dysmenorrhea by helping in the relaxation of the muscles of the uterus.	Calcium: 750 mg twice a day Magnesium: 500 mg twice a day
Evening primrose oil or Starflower oil	These supplements are high in omega-6 fatty acids, which are converted in the body to anti-inflammatory prostaglandins, which may neutralize the effect of the inflammatory prostaglandins that are a possible cause of dysmenorrhea.	Evening primrose oil: 1 g three times a day Starflower oil: 500 mg three times a day

6

HEAVY PERIODS

Heavy periods can be a debilitating problem for a significant number of women. Excessive blood loss can quite quickly lead to iron-deficiency anemia, so it is important that you have this checked by your doctor. Interestingly, iron deficiency can be a cause, as well as a consequence, of heavy periods. This means that extra iron may actually help to reduce blood loss in addition to correcting the anemia. See Anemia (page 80) for advice on dietary measures to combat iron deficiency.

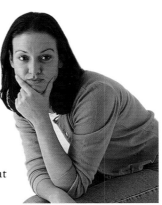

Warning

High doses of vitamin A are not suitable for extended use. Pregnant women and women planning pregnancy are advised not to take more than 10,000 IU of vitamin A each day in supplement form.

WHAT IS A HEAVY PERIOD?

Average blood loss during menstruation is 4 tablespoons (60 ml), but there is enormous variation between women. A woman is usually dignosed as having menorrhagia if blood loss is more than 6 tablespoons (90 ml) each period. In practical terms this means significant bleeding that continues for longer than seven days or if bleeding is so severe that normal sanitary protection is inadequate.

USEFUL SUPPLEMENTS FOR HEAVY PERIODS

Supplement	Action	Dose
Iron	Take supplements only if a deficiency has been established by your doctor.	50–100 mg a day
Vitamin A	It is thought that high-dose vitamin A works by changing female hormone balance. You should notice a reduction in your menstrual flow within two or three periods. Do not take more than 10,000 IU of vitamin A a day if you are pregnant or planning pregnancy.	50,000–75,000 IU a day for four to six weeks. Then 10,000–25,000 IU a day

6

PREMENSTRUAL SYNDROME

Premenstrual syndrome (PMS) is a term used to describe a combination of physical and mental symptoms that may occur in the week or two prior to menstruation. Typical features of PMS include irritability, depression, tearfulness, fatigue, food cravings, abdominal bloating, breast tenderness, fluid retention, and weight gain. The condition is highly individual, with the exact blend of symptoms and their duration varying enormously between women.

WHAT CAUSES PMS?

PMS is due to hormonal fluctuations in the second half of the menstrual cycle and is thought to affect 80 percent of women to some degree. The conventional medical approach is centered around symptom relief, such as diuretics for fluid retention, or the use of the oral contraceptive pill. However, many studies have shown that PMS can be very successfully treated with certain lifestyle changes and nutritional supplements.

ADJUSTING YOUR DIET

Sugar, caffeine, and alcohol all seem to increase the severity of PMS, and it makes sense to avoid foods and drinks containing these items, especially in the second half of your cycle. Women who eat a low-fat, high-fiber diet seem to have a reduced risk of PMS – so eat a diet low in red meat and dairy products but high in fruits, vegetables, and whole grains. Foods rich in B vitamins, magnesium, and vitamin E, such as whole grains and seeds, seem to be particularly beneficial.

FOOD CRAVINGS

Food cravings, particularly for sweet and starchy food, are a feature of PMS in some women. Such cravings tend to be caused by fluctuations in blood sugar that occur in the premenstrual phase. To prevent the blood sugar level from dropping too low, it is important to eat regularly and to base the diet around foods that give a sustained release of sugar into the bloodstream, including meat, fish, fresh vegetables, and whole-grain starches like whole-wheat bread, brown rice, and whole-wheat pasta. Chromium is a useful supplement if you suffer from this problem. It helps to combat cravings by regulating blood sugar levels. Take 200–400 mcg a day.

6

EXERCISE TO COMBAT PMS

Another lifestyle factor that is well known to reduce the symptoms of PMS in the long term is exercise. Try to get about half an hour's exercise such as jogging, aerobics, cycling, or swimming on most days. If you have not been used to taking regular exercise, start with brisk walking, and graduate to more demanding exercise after a few weeks.

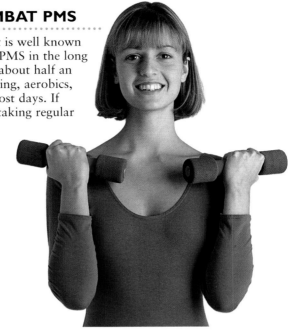

Warning

Excessive intake of vitamin B₆ can have an adverse effect on the nervous system. Do not exceed the recommended dose.

USEFUL SUPPLEMENTS

Supplement	Action	Dose
Vitamin B₆	B₆ has been found to help a significant proportion of women with PMS and appears to affect the whole range of potential symptoms. Take 50 mg each day, increasing this dose to a daily maximum of 150 mg, if necessary, in the premenstrual phase. In addition, take a B-complex supplement each day to make sure the level of B vitamins in your body stays in balance.	50 mg one to three times a day
Magnesium	This nutrient is commonly deficient in young women. Additional quantities may help relieve PMS, including painful periods.	400 mg a day
Evening primrose oil or **Starflower oil**	These supplements are high in omega-6 fatty acids that help to maintain hormonal balance in the body.	1 g three times a day or 500 mg three times a day

6

LUMPY BREASTS

Lumpiness of the breasts that is often associated with pain and discomfort before a period is known as fibrocystic breast disease (FBD). It is caused by the presence of multiple cysts (fluid-filled sacs) in the breasts. This condition is thought to affect about 30 percent of premenopausal women. While the precise cause of the condition is unclear, there does seem to be some evidence that it is linked to an excess of the hormone estrogen in the body.

FOOD FACTORS

The symptoms of fibrocystic breast disease seem to be made worse by the consumption of caffeine and caffeinelike substances found in coffee, tea, cola, and chocolate. One study showed an improvement in virtually every woman who abstained from these foodstuffs. Herb and fruit teas and barley and chicory-based coffee substitutes are much healthier.

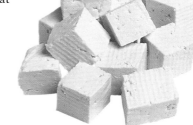

To make sure you receive all the nutrients you need for healthy hormone balance in the body, eat a diet based on whole, unprocessed foods such as whole-wheat bread, brown rice, fresh vegetables, fruits, beans, legumes, nuts, and seeds. In addition, you may get benefit from eating more soy-based products such as tofu which contain plant hormones that seem to block the effect of estrogen in the body (see below).

THE HORMONELIKE EFFECTS OF SOYBEANS

It is interesting to note that the breast cancer rate in the West is roughly four times that in Japan. One consistent dietary difference between these two cultures is the intake of soy-based foods. The majority of breast cancers are what is termed "hormone dependent," which means that hormones such as estrogen play an important part in their development. Soy foods contain substances called isoflavones, which appear to have the ability to block the effect of estrogen on breast cancer cells, thereby slowing down or inactivating estrogen. The recommended dose of isoflavones is 40 mg a day. To get this amount, you would need to drink a cup of soy milk daily or consume about 3–4 ounces (100 g) of tofu.

6

BREAST CANCER PREVENTION

Breast cancer is the leading cause of cancer death in women, so it is important for every woman to take sensible precautions to lessen the risk of developing the disease, and to be alert for symptoms that may indicate a problem.

■ Breast cancer seems to be associated with a high-fat, low-fiber diet. So base your diet around high-fiber, low-fat foods such as fresh fruits, vegetables, and whole grains like brown rice, whole-wheat bread, and whole-wheat pasta.

■ Be familar with the appearance of your breasts and the normal cyclical changes in size and shape.

■ Seek prompt medical advice if you notice any new lumps, discharge from a nipple, inversion of the nipple, or unusual puckering of the skin of the breast.

■ Some types of breast cancer seem to have a strong genetic basis. If a close family member has suffered from the disease, discuss this with your doctor, who may arrange for special monitoring.

Warning

Although the cysts that cause the lumpiness in FBD are benign (non-cancerous), any woman with a lump or lumps in her breast should have this assessed by her doctor.

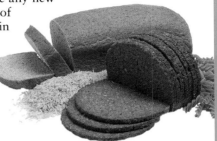

USEFUL SUPPLEMENTS

Supplement	Action	Dose
Vitamin E	Studies show that vitamin E can be very effective in relieving the symptoms of FBD, perhaps by helping to balance hormone levels in the body. If there is any history of high blood pressure, the dose of vitamin E should be built up gradually over several weeks.	400–800 IU a day
Evening primrose oil or Starflower oil	Many women find these supplements help to relieve the discomfort of FBD. This may be due to the hormone-regulating and anti-inflammatory actions of these oils.	1 g three times a day 500 mg three times a day

6

YEAST INFECTIONS

Vaginal yeast infection or "thrush" is caused by the overgrowth of a yeast organism known as *Candida albicans*. Typical symptoms of this condition include a thick, white, cottage cheeselike discharge from the vagina and/or vaginal itching and irritation. There may also be discomfort when passing urine. The overgrowth of yeast in the body is linked to certain factors. One of the most common features in thrush is the use of antibiotics.

HOW ANTIBIOTICS CAUSE THRUSH

While antibiotics may kill unhealthy bacteria in the body, they may also kill many of the healthy bacteria in the intestinal tract that are responsible for keeping yeast organisms in check. Recurrent courses of antibiotics throughout life can disturb the natural balance of organisms in the gut, and therefore the vagina, leading to yeast overgrowth. Other factors that seem to predispose to thrush infection are the oral contraceptive pill, stress, and a diet high in sugar, refined carbohydrates, yeast, and alcohol.

RECURRING THRUSH

The conventional medical approach to thrush is generally to use antifungal creams or pessaries to treat the infection. However, despite these measures, many women find that they suffer from chronic, relapsing bouts of thrush. The reason for this is because the reservoir for candida in the body is actually the digestive tract, so treating only the vaginal source of the infection will not usually bring lasting relief.

FOODS TO AVOID

In the digestive tract, candida thrives on certain foods:

■ Sugar, refined carbohydrates (white bread, white rice, pasta).

■ Yeasty, moldy, or fermented foods such as bread, yeast extract, stock cubes and gravy mixes, soy sauce, vinegar, cheese.

■ Alcohol.

■ Peanuts and mushrooms.

Eliminate all the above foods from your diet for at least two months.

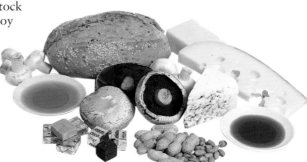

FOODS THAT COMBAT YEAST INFECTION

A diet based around fresh vegetables, brown rice, meat, fish, beans, and legumes, together with plenty of water and herb teas, will help starve candida out of the system. Natural live yogurt taken every day can help to replenish healthy bacteria in the gut and restore a healthy balance of organisms.

HYGIENE

To help prevent infection and to hasten recovery, protect the natural acidity of the vagina. Do not douche or use soaps or deodorants in the genital area. Washing the external genital area with plain water is adequate.

USEFUL SUPPLEMENTS

Supplement	Action	Dose
Acidophilus	To help restore a healthy balance of organisms in the gut, it is a good idea to take a supplement containing healthy gut bacteria such as acidophilus. Take this for two months. This supplement should be kept refrigerated. Acidophilus capsules can also be inserted into the vagina for local relief from the symptoms of thrush.	1–10 billion live organisms a day
Milk thistle	Long-standing yeast infection in the digestive tract tends to stress the liver through the production of toxins. Milk thistle can help strengthen the liver and prevent toxicity in the body as a whole.	100–150 mg three times a day
Caprylic acid	This extract of coconut is known to have antifungal activity. Do not take this supplement if you are pregnant or planning pregnancy.	400–500 mg three times a day
Tea tree oil	Tea tree oil can be very effective in treating vaginal yeast infections. A solution of the oil can be made with water, and a tampon can be soaked in the solution and then inserted into the vagina.	

6

CERVICAL PROBLEMS

In a small but significant number of women, the cells of the cervix may undergo certain changes that are known as "cervical intraepithial neoplasia" (CIN). CIN is classified according to its severity. CIN1, CIN2, and CIN3 denote mild, moderate, and severe degrees of abnormality respectively. If CIN is allowed to progress unchecked, it will ultimately develop into early localized cancer (called carcinoma *in situ*) and then finally full-blown cervical cancer.

MEDICAL TREATMENTS

Any woman found to have CIN will normally be advised to have a repeat smear or an examination of the cervix with a viewing instrument (colposcopy). During colposcopy, samples of tissue are sometimes removed (biopsy) or the affected area is treated with laser or electrocoagulation (both of which use heat to destroy abnormal tissue) or cryosurgery (which uses cold to destroy tissue).

THE RISK FACTORS

■ Cervical abnormalities are more common in women who have had a large number of sexual partners. However, some women develop abnormal cervical cells despite having only one or a small number of sexual partners.

■ The risk is increased if there has been contact with the virus that causes genital warts. Using condoms during intercourse may reduce your risk in the long term.

■ Smoking increases the risk of CIN, so if you are a smoker you should stop or at least cut down. There is also an increased risk if your regular partner smokes, so he should be encouraged to give up, too.

CERVICAL SCREENING

The early stages of cervical cancer are symptomless. Adult women are therefore advised to have regular cervical checks by means of a cervical smear test. This should be done on a regular basis between the ages of 21 and 64. The test involves taking a sample of cells from the cervix and examining them for abnormalities under a microscope.

Warning

Even if you have been having regular cervical screening, seek medical advice if you notice a blood-stained discharge between periods or after menopause, or if you experience bleeding after intercourse.

ANTIOXIDANT SUPPORT

Studies show that cervical dysplasia is associated with low levels of the antioxidant nutrients betacarotene, vitamins A, C, and E, and the mineral selenium. Make sure you eat a healthful diet that contains plenty of fresh fruits, vegetables, seeds, nuts, and whole grains to make sure you receive adequate amounts of these nutrients.

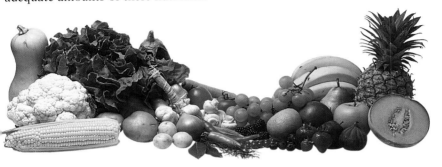

USEFUL SUPPLEMENTS

Supplement	Action	Dose
Folic acid	One nutrient that seems to be of particular benefit in correcting CIN is folic acid. Very high doses of this vitamin have been shown to improve abnormal smears in some women. Take for three months. Because folic acid can mask the signs of B_{12} deficiency, a B_{12} supplement of this vitamin should be taken each day, too.	5 mg, twice a day
Antioxidant formulation	Additional antioxidants may help prevent and even reverse the processes that cause abnormal cervical cells. Look for a formulation that contains betacarotene, vitamins A, C, and E, and the mineral selenium.	Follow the instructions on the label
Lycopene	A high intake of this relative of beta-carotene – which is derived mainly from tomatoes – is associated with a reduced risk of developing CIN.	10 mg a day

6

PREGNANCY SUPPORT

There is no doubt that the nutritional status of the mother and father at the time of conception has an important impact on the health of the ensuing pregnancy. What is also clear is that the level of certain nutrients in the mother's diet during pregnancy has a tremendous bearing on the health of the baby at birth and throughout the first few months of life. This means, of course, that good nutrition is of the utmost importance both before and during pregnancy.

PREPARING FOR CONCEPTION

Ideally, you should prepare for pregnancy some months before you anticipate becoming pregnant. Both you and your partner should eat a healthful nutritious diet based on whole, unprocessed foods such as poultry, fish, fresh fruits and vegetables, nuts, seeds, beans and legumes, and whole grains such as whole-wheat bread, whole-wheat pasta, and brown rice.

SAFEGUARDING YOUR BABY

It is a good idea to abstain from alcohol for three months prior to conception and during the whole of the pregnancy. Excessive consumption of alcohol during pregnancy can lead to a condition known as "fetal alcohol syndrome," which can result in mental retardation, brain, heart, and nervous system problems, and facial abnormalities. Caffeine should also be avoided before and during pregnancy, since the consumption of caffeine is actually linked to problems with fertility and increased risk of miscarriage. Continue to eat the same healthful diet as recommended for preparing for conception to make sure you and your baby receive all the nutrients you need.

Warning

Pregnant women should not take more than 10,000 IU of vitamin A a day in supplement form, since there is some evidence that this may increase the risk of fetal abnormalities.

6

PREVENTING NEURAL TUBE DEFECTS

About three in 2,000 babies are born with an abnormality of the brain or spinal cord which doctors refer to as "neural tube defects" (NTDs). The most common type of NTD is a condition called spina bifida, where one or more bones of the spinal column do not form properly and fail to protect the spinal cord. The risk of NTDs is substantially reduced if the mother takes supplements of folic acid. Folic acid supplementation also seems to improve a baby's birth weight and reduce the risk of infection in the mother. Ideally, you should take 400 mcg of folic acid from at least three months before conceiving and during the first three months of pregnancy.

Dark green vegetables are a key source of folic acid in the diet.

IRON SUPPLEMENTS

Many women become somewhat anemic during pregnancy. In the past pregnant women were routinely given iron supplements to prevent this. Research has now shown that slight anemia is not harmful to the mother or baby and iron supplements are usually recommended only if anemia is severe.

USEFUL SUPPLEMENTS

Supplement	Action	Dose
Multivitamin and mineral preparation for pregnancy	It can be beneficial to take a supplement that has been specifically formulated for use during pregnancy. Nutrients that seem to be of particular benefit during pregnancy include vitamins B_1 and B_3. Supplementation with these nutrients is associated with increased weight and size of newborn infants. Another important nutrient is calcium, since the body's requirement for this mineral doubles during pregnancy. Ideally, you should start taking this supplement three months prior to conception.	Follow the instructions on the label
Folic acid	Folic acid helps to prevent neural tube defects. If you have previously had a baby with this problem, a higher dose may be recommended.	400 mcg a day

6

MORNING SICKNESS

Morning sickness is a common problem that usually starts before the sixth week of pregnancy and disappears by the twelfth week. Although morning sickness is almost always harmless, any woman who is experiencing severe or prolonged problems should consult her doctor. The nausea and vomiting in early pregnancy invariably cause discomfort and distress for sufferers, but simple natural remedies can often be very effective in bringing symptoms under control. Other digestive problems are also common in pregnancy, notably heartburn and constipation.

COMBATING MORNING SICKNESS

■ Cut down on fatty foods such as red meat, dairy products, and fried foods, which tend to make the feeling of sickness worse.

■ Another good idea is to eat small meals (including breakfast) quite often during the day. This helps to reduce the load on the digestive tract and can help maintain a stable level of sugar in the bloodstream. Blood sugar fluctuations are a common feature in morning sickness.

■ One natural and effective remedy for morning sickness is ginger. Chewing a piece of gingerroot throughout the day or drinking ginger tea made from grated or sliced gingerroot may help relieve your symptoms quite quickly.

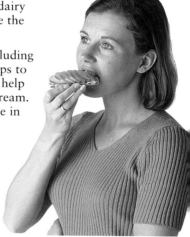

USEFUL SUPPLEMENTS

Supplement	Action	Dose
Ginger	Ginger capsules are a convenient form in which to take this traditional remedy.	250 mg three or four times a day
Vitamin B_6	B_6 is another natural substance known to help women suffering from nausea in pregnancy.	50 mg once or twice a day

6

MENOPAUSE

During her reproductive years, a woman's cycle is regulated by a variety of hormones, the most important of which are estrogen and progesterone. Around the time of menopause, the production of these hormones drops dramatically, which can give rise to a number of symptoms including night sweats, hot flashes, vaginal dryness, mood disturbance, and loss of libido. Often, many of these symptoms resolve themselves once the hormonal turmoil of menopause is over. However, in some women, symptoms may persist for many years.

HORMONE REPLACEMENT THERAPY

The conventional medical approach to such menopausal symptoms is hormone replacement therapy (HRT). This can be effective, particularly for hot flashes, while other added benefits are said to be a reduction in risk of both heart disease and osteoporosis. Recent evidence suggests that the effect of HRT on heart disease is not as great as was first thought, and any bone-protective effect is lost once the medication is discontinued. What is more, there is evidence that HRT may increase the risk of certain cancers such as breast cancer. Taking better care of your general health around the time of menopause can reduce the need for HRT. In particular, cut down on the amount of saturated (animal) fats in the diet and eat plenty of fresh vegetables and fruits, beans, whole grains, seeds, and nuts.

POSTMENOPAUSAL PROTECTION FOR BONES

Because osteoporosis is a particular problem after the time of menopause, menopausal women should increase their intake of foods that are rich in calcium and magnesium, both of which are essential for healthy bone formation. Green leafy vegetables, sardines, mackerel, seafood, and sesame seeds are all good sources of these essential minerals (see also page 61).

USEFUL SUPPLEMENT

Supplement	Action	Dose
Vitamin E	Clinical studies have shown that vitamin E can be very effective in relieving hot flashes and vaginal dryness in menopausal women.	400 IU twice a day, reduced to 200 IU twice a day when symptoms are controlled

6

INDEX

ACKNOWLEDGMENTS

The author and the publishers gratefully acknowledge the invaluable contribution made by Laura Wickenden who took all the photographs in this book except:

16 top Paul Bricknell; 21 middle Iain Bagwell; 23 bottom Iain Bagwell; 27 top ZEFA/Power Stock; 33 David de Lossy/The Image Bank; 39 bottom left John Gerlach/Earth Scenes/Oxford Scientific Films; 39 bottom right Iain Bagwell; 48 top ZEFA/Power Stock; 69 top Stephen Marks/ The Image Bank.